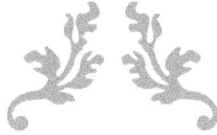

FIBER FUELED: THE PLANT-BASED EATING, HEALTHY GUT 101

Restore Your Health with a Microbiome Diet—Natural Weight-loss Journey of Feeding Yourself
Fuller with Brain Food Dietary, Intelligent Nutrients

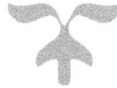

Edyth J. Garson

Contents

Now It Begins

"To eat is a necessity, but to eat intelligently is an art."—**La Rochefoucauld**

Do you know how the sense of taste develops? If it is innate or not? And in what way does it influence the choice of food? And why do we like some flavors more than others? Another aspect that should be noted is that obese people have altered sensitivity to this sense, and it differs from people with a normal BMI.

And have you ever wondered why, depending on our mood, does our appetite increase or decrease? Do we have a predilection for consuming certain foods? And finally, do you know that personality also plays a role in our food choices? All these questions are the ones that several authors have tried to solve through studies and reviews that exist in this regard. I think it is a fascinating topic.

Flavor perception is real.

First of all, you should know that the ability to perceive flavors begins in the uterus as the taste system begins to develop (the cells that perceive it are formed and are functional from the first trimester of gestation and reach their maturity in the second trimester) and smell.

It is also known that the two senses mentioned above are fundamental in the development of food preferences, which are genetic but also the result of the interaction between environmental, social, and biological factors. These preferences can vary throughout life. Only those that are innate are maintained until childhood and decrease from adolescence.

Also, depending on the taste, some responses or others are produced. For example, the sweet taste and umami (5th characteristic flavor of soy sauce and Chinese food-related to an increase in BMI) generate positive responses. In contrast, sour and bitter flavors generate negative responses. At the individual level, we have genes related to the senses of sweet, umami, and bitter, so the sensitivity to them is different. Greater sensitivity to bitter means a greater perception of the sweet. The bitter taste is perceived through the TAS2R38 gene (associated with healthy eating in women), and it has also been seen that children who have it have a greater preference for sweet foods and drinks. Studies on the perception of bitterness have found a relationship with an increased risk of alcoholism.

And how does the development of taste occur? The fetus inside the mother's womb can inhale and swallow a part of the amniotic fluid that contains amino acids and glucose that come from the mother's diet and the environment in which it is found. Several studies indicate that the injection of a sweet taste in the amniotic fluid stimulates the fetus to swallow. In contrast, the bitter one produces the opposite effect. Even studies in premature infants show that offering a solution of glucose or sucrose results in increased suction.

On the other hand, lemon stimulates salivation. It should be considered that at the age between 2 and 5 years, adaptive behavior occurs due to the introduction of food known as neophobia and is characterized by a refusal to eat new foods. This is due to the influence of experience and familiarity. And how can you get them to try it? It is nothing more than repeated exposure to that food (6-15 times) without forcing the situation since the rejection can increase and continue throughout life. Another thing that is not convenient to do is restrict food since what is achieved is to increase the desire to eat it. So the best solution is by setting an example, that is, for the child to see that we eat it without problems.

There are changes in the preference of tastes throughout life since in adults, it depends on age, sex, health, education, and income, and also, it has been observed that the consumption of healthy food increases with age. Another aspect to consider is that from old age, the perception of taste and smell decreases.

Choice of food tells a lot about you.

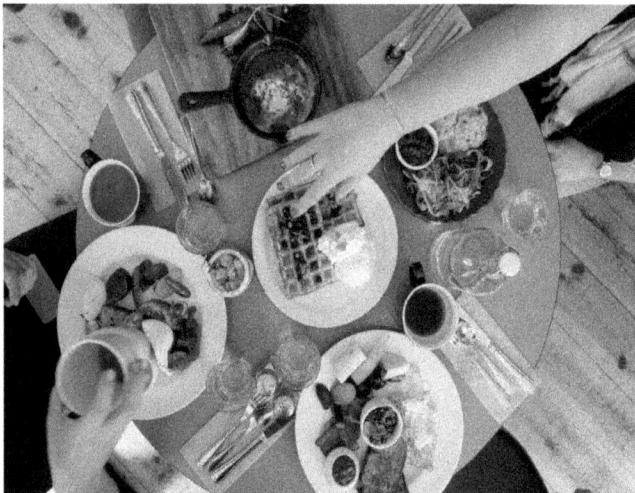

And in what way do we choose food? Food choice is conditioned by the availability of food, mood, environment, health, allergies, comfort, appetite, price, habits, culture, and sensory characteristics (color, taste, and aroma) and influences eating behavior.

As for the sensitivity of taste, it differs between people. For this reason, a clinical trial was conducted on the variation in the perception of taste in obese and people with a normal BMI. It was assessed utilizing strips with flavors (sweet, acid, bitter, umami, salty, and neutral) at different concentrations. They first had to identify the taste and subsequently rate it according to concentration. The results indicate that obese people were less sensitive to salty, umami, and bitter tastes. Also, the older it is, the easier it is to identify flavors correctly. It was the same with women.

Emotions also influence intake. They have observed that during periods of stress, there is an increase in caloric foods rich in fat and sugar (sweets and chocolate). In university, students eat an unhealthy diet or increase the calories in the diet during exams or stress, which means a greater tendency to follow weight loss diets or restrict certain foods' consumption. It has also been observed that depression prevents healthy eating and involves skipping some meals of the day.

The effect of macronutrients (carbohydrates, proteins, and fats) on mood has also been assessed. Carbohydrates generate a state of calm and drowsiness, so an increase in their intake supposes a lower risk of depression, but proteins increase. Instead, fats cause fatigue and reduce alertness and attention. These results indicate that mood affects food choices and vice versa.

And finally, I would like to comment on how personality influences the choice of food. It is conditioned by environmental, socio-cultural, and economic factors and knowledge about food (nutrients they contain, how to cook them, and where to buy them), and interpersonal relationships.

There are five types of personality:

- Emotional instability (tendency to depression, hostility, and nervousness). It is related to the low quality of the diet due to comfort.

- Be outgoing (active and optimistic person)

- Meticulousness (strong, orderly, and disciplined). It has been linked to practicing physical exercise and avoiding risky behaviors (abusing alcohol, not using seat belts, and smoking).

- Kindness (sympathy and being altruistic)

- Open to new experiences (they are curious and imaginative). It is related to a healthy diet based on the consumption of fruits, vegetables, cereals, dairy products, fish, the Mediterranean diet, and lower meat consumption. It means lower consumption of canned foods, sausages, mashed potatoes, cookies, chocolate, puddings, etc.

Varies based on gender. Women score higher on conscientiousness, emotional instability, and kindness. In contrast, men are characterized by being more outgoing and open to new experiences.

Food is essential to have a good quality of life. However, there is a determining factor when choosing what to eat: personality. In this way, eating habits vary. A calm person does not consume the same as those who are more active.

The impulsive eater.

Those people who are characterized by having this type of personality can be hyperactive and easily distracted. In this way, they may fall before some 'temptations' due to the anxiety they feel at times.

Food is included in this order of ideas. The impulsive tend to resort to junk food and packages, as they are those products that have a closer range.

Insurance.

These people are more organized and punctual. Therefore, they can be adapted more easily to eating plans, diets, and change their habits more easily. Likewise, they would achieve easier weight loss and attend a gym with discipline.

Constant mood swings.

Some people have highly variable emotions, which means that they can have very positive or very negative reactions at certain times. Likewise, it influences the diet. The more changeable someone is, the more they will eat.

Therefore, it is appropriate to recognize this instability, and learn to eat more balanced, complementing it with an exercise routine.

Extroverts also have it differently.

More open people may accumulate more stress and consume high amounts of calories, which will lead them to gain weight more easily.

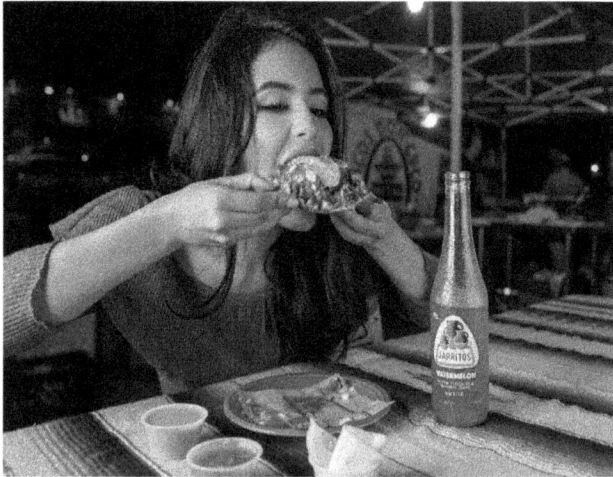

Early risers versus night owls.

Some people perform better at night than in the morning. Despite this, those who stay up late are more likely to consume additional calories, mostly from foods rich in fat. In other words, night owls can gain more weight.

For their part, those who are more productive in the morning have a lower risk of being overweight since they have rested better, which favors a correct diet.

It should be remembered that expert recommendations indicate that you should sleep between seven and nine hours at night.

Egocentric as it gets.

If someone's goal is to lose weight, a self-centered person will have a better chance of achieving it because they consider their interests more and are more willing to choose what to eat.

On the other hand, those who care about pleasing others may be more interested in them than in themselves. For example, they may meet up with their friends to go to exercise or do other activities.

#MakeTheShift.

Chapter 1: The Easiest Guide to Nutrition

As the eBook title suggests, this book will also incorporate food choices and items which may not be plant-based. While I thoroughly profess to make the shift, I would still prefer to respect personal choices that are contradictory. Remember: there is power in coexistence.

Nutrition is a relatively young science, with enormous difficulties. Until recently, the tools to understand the effect of different nutrients on the human body and health were very limited.

The normal thing was to study human groups that ate more or less the same. They looked for differences over time, which invites other factors (exercise, tobacco, and alcohol consumption, genetics) to influence the results. Or volunteers were locked up in a hospital, and what they ate was monitored to the millimeter and expensive and uncomfortable procedure.

The most important studies that determined the late twentieth century's nutritional recommendations were population studies, with the disadvantage that it is not possible to establish a clear cause-and-effect relationship. That, when the interests of the food industry did not manipulate them.

To date, most of the studies are still population-based and establish correlations, not causes. Studies with laboratory mice are very comprehensive, but humans behave differently in nine out of ten cases. However, there are relatively new techniques such as **radioisotope tracers and stable isotopes** that allow "following" the components of food on their journey through the human body, without the need to vivisect volunteers.

Yet decades of ups and downs have led to great confusion among the public, who, with the mainstream media's collaboration and their penchant for exaggerated headlines, are often met with contradictory statements. "Coffee is dangerous." "Coffee is healthy." "Fats make you fat." "Carbohydrates make you fat." So, ad infinitum.

This is a list of minimal, nutritional principles that most studies and experts agree on:

Sugar is a bad idea

Almost all processed foods contain sugar in one form or another. You will find sugar in your skimmed yogurts or with supposedly healthy bifidobacterial, in your sauces, batters, cookies, and of course, in large quantities in industrial pastries and sugary soft drinks. It does not matter if refined sugar, cane sugar, corn syrup, fruit juice concentrate, or even honey. The basic chemical composition is the same in all cases and the effects on your body as well. Excess sugar, especially from beverages and especially in children, is directly related to obesity, coronary heart disease, and type 2 diabetes.

Common sugar and almost all substitutes are half fructose. Fructose is metabolized in the liver as it cannot be used directly by cells. All that fructose causes fatty liver, increased visceral fat, and insulin resistance.

Trans fats are bad

The artificially obtained trans fats and that you will find on your food labels as "partially hydrogenated vegetable fats" have not yet been banned by the European Union. However, they have been banned by Denmark and the US, among other countries, and it is about time that they were eliminated from everyone's diet. These fats replace butter and other solid fats, especially in industrial pastries, cookies, sauces, or pre-cooked foods. They increase abdominal fat, cause insulin resistance, and therefore long-term diabetes. Chronic inflammation and mortality from cardiovascular diseases increase. Come on, a gem of food.

Eating more vegetables is healthy

No matter what type of diet you follow, increasing your intake of vegetables has beneficial effects on your health. Vegetables, vegetables, legumes, and mushrooms contain minerals, vitamins, fiber, and other compounds such as antioxidants and enzymes whose effects are becoming known. In a controlled study (the most reliable), it has been seen that increasing the intake of vegetables and fruits lowers blood pressure and increases antioxidants in the blood. Population studies in the US indicate that the people who consume the most vegetables and fruits have type 2 diabetes the least.

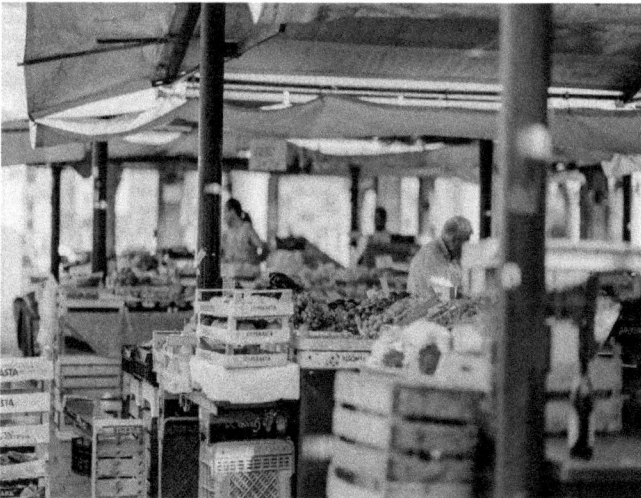

Vitamin D deficiency is widespread and harmful

Vitamin D is special because it behaves like a hormone in your body. It is also so because, unlike other vitamins, the body can produce it when the skin is exposed to the sun's ultraviolet rays. However, many people live in climates where it is not possible to expose themselves to the sun, and when they do, the risk of skin cancer forces them to use sunscreen, which prevents the generation of vitamin D.

Unfortunately, it is difficult to get vitamin D from the diet, and this is a problem. Lack of vitamin D increases the risk of heart attack and osteoporosis. In turn, vitamin D prevents different types of cancer. One solution is to take a vitamin D supplement, or as in the old days, a tablespoon of cod liver oil a day.

You need to take omega-3 fats

Omega-3 fatty acids are essential for your body to function properly. There are three main ones: alpha-linolenic acid (ALA) that is extracted from plants, and eicosatetraenoic (EPA) and docosahexaenoic (DHA) acids that are obtained mainly from animals, especially from oily fish, although it is also found in omega-3 fortified eggs and milk and grass-raised meat.

ALA from plants is not directly usable by the human body and has to be transformed into DHA or EPA. Still, this conversion is very inefficient, so it is difficult to achieve adequate levels of omega-3 only with plant sources. Omega-3 deficiency causes depression, affects cognitive abilities, and increases the risk of cardiovascular **disease**. Not surprisingly, your brain is made up of 20% DHA.

Refined seed oils are unhealthy

Refined soybean, corn, rapeseed, or sunflower oils are unnatural. Just as olive oil has been known for millennia and is easy to extract, high pressures and temperatures are applied to extract the oil from these seeds, making them unstable and easily oxidized. These oils are rich in omega-6 polyunsaturated fatty acids, which have an inflammatory effect.

When the percentage of omega-6 fats increases and that of omega-3 (anti-inflammatory) decreases, the risk of obesity and cardiovascular disease increases, the excess of omega-6 also increases oxidative stress, responsible for many chronic diseases and cancers, and contrary to what was believed, increases oxidized LDL cholesterol, which is implicated in cardiovascular diseases.

Low-fat diets do not prevent cardiovascular disease or obesity

For decades the idea has been propagated that a low-fat diet is the healthiest, with a maximum of 10-15% of total calories each day coming from fat. This diet was supposed to be the right one to fight obesity and cardiovascular disease; today's consensus is the opposite.

Your body can get energy from fat or carbohydrates, so low-fat diets are necessarily rich in carbohydrates, especially starch (flour, rice, etc.) and sugar. However, it is proven that excess carbohydrates are not well tolerated for people **with insulin resistance**, such as obese people, or even worse, those with type 2 diabetes. In one study, diabetic patients were given a ketogenic diet, very low in carbohydrates and high in fat for six months. The result was that **95% of them were able to reduce or eliminate their** diabetes **medication**. After examining the most rigorous controlled studies, **there is no evidence that** low-fat diets reduce cardiovascular disease risk.

What is all this based on?

The relation between consumption of sugar-sweetened drinks and childhood obesity: a prospective, observational analysis: a study by National Library of Medicine.

For each additional serving of sugar-sweetened beverage consumed, both the body mass index (BMI) and the frequency of obesity increased after adjustment for anthropometric, demographic, dietary, and lifestyle variables. Initial consumption of sugar-sweetened beverages was also independently associated with the change in BMI.

Consuming fructose-sweetened, not glucose-sweetened beverages, increases visceral adiposity and lipids and decreases insulin sensitivity in overweight/obese humans: a study by National Library of Medicine. These data suggest that dietary fructose specifically increases de novo lipogenesis, promotes dyslipidemia, decreases insulin sensitivity, and increases visceral adiposity in overweight/obese adults.

Trans fat diet induces abdominal obesity and changes in insulin sensitivity in monkeys – a study by National Library of Medicine. Under controlled eating conditions, long-term trans-fat consumption was an independent factor in weight gain. Trans fats increased intra-abdominal fat deposition, even in the absence of excess calories, and were associated with insulin resistance, with evidence that there is an alteration in the transduction of the insulin receptor binding signal.

Dietary intake of trans fatty acids and systemic inflammation in womena study by National Library of Medicine. The consumption of trans fats is positively associated with markers of systemic inflammation in women. Further investigation of the influences of trans fats on inflammation and the implications for coronary heart disease, diabetes, and other conditions is warranted.

Intake of saturated and trans unsaturated fatty acids and risk of all cause mortality, cardiovascular disease, and type 2 diabetes: systematic review and meta-analysis of observational studies: a study by National Library of Medicine. Trans fats are associated with all-cause mortality, total CHD, and CHD mortality, probably due to higher industrial trans-fat intake levels than ruminant trans fats.

Effects of fruit and vegetable consumption on plasma antioxidant concentrations and blood pressure: a randomized controlled trial: a study by National Library of Medicine. The effects of the intervention on the consumption of fruits and vegetables, plasma antioxidants, and blood pressure are expected to reduce cardiovascular disease in the general population.

Fruit and Vegetable Consumption and Diabetes Mellitus Incidence among US Adults: a ScienceDirect study. The intake of fruits and vegetables may be inversely related to the incidence of diabetes, especially among women. Education may partly explain this association.

25-hydroxyvitamin D and risk of myocardial infarction in men: a prospective study: a study by National Library of Medicine. Low levels of 25 (OH) D are associated with a graded increased risk of myocardial infarction, even after controlling for factors known to be associated with coronary artery disease.

Fracture prevention with vitamin D supplementation: a meta-analysis of randomized controlled trials: a study by National Library of Medicine. Oral administration of vitamin D supplements between 700 and 800 IU/d appears to reduce the risk of hip fractures and any nonvertebral fracture in outpatient or institutionalized older people. An oral dose of vitamin D of 400 IU / d is not sufficient to prevent fractures.

Vitamin D and calcium supplementation reduce cancer risk: results of a randomized trial: a study by National Library of Medicine. Improving the nutritional status of calcium and vitamin D substantially reduces the risk of cancer in postmenopausal women.

An Increase in the Omega-6 / Omega-3 Fatty Acid Ratio Increases the Risk for Obesity: a study by National Library of Medicine. Recent studies in humans show that in addition to absolute amounts of omega-6 and omega-3 fatty acid intake, the omega-6 / omega-3 ratio plays an important role in increasing the development of obesity

n-6 fatty acid-specific. Mixed polyunsaturated dietary interventions have different effects on CHD risk: a meta-analysis of randomized controlled trials: a study by National Library of Medicine. Advice to specifically increase n-6 PUFA intake, based on pooled data from n-3 / n-6 controlled studies, is unlikely to provide the expected benefits and may increase cardiovascular disease risks and mortality.

Lowering dietary linoleic acid reduces bioactive oxidized linoleic acid metabolites in humans: a study by National Library of Medicine. These results show that decreasing dietary linoleic acid can reduce the synthesis and accumulation of oxidized linoleic acid derivatives implicated in various pathological conditions.

Changes in Dietary Fat Intake Alter Plasma Levels of Oxidized Low-Density Lipoprotein and Lipoprotein (a): a research by AHA Journals. In conclusion, we found that a diet traditionally considered antiatherogenic (low in saturated fat and high in polyunsaturated fat and natural antioxidants) increased plasma levels of LDL and Circulating oxidized lp (a).

The health benefits of omega-3 polyunsaturated fatty acids: a review of the evidence: a study by National Library of Medicine. Most of the intervention studies, which found associations between various conditions and the intake of fish oils or their derivatives, used n-3 intakes well above the 0.2 g day recommended by the Committee on Medical Aspects of Food Policy (EAT).

The effect of a low-carbohydrate, ketogenic diet versus a low-glycemic index diet on glycemic control in type 2 diabetes mellitus Diabetes: a study by National Library of Medicine. medications was reduced or eliminated in 95.2% of the low-carbohydrate ketogenic diet vs. 62% of participants on a low-calorie, low-glycemic diet.

Evidence from randomized controlled trials does not support current dietary fat guidelines: a systematic review and meta-analysis: a study by National Library of Medicine. The currently available evidence found no significant difference in all-cause mortality or coronary disease mortality due to dietary fat interventions. Currently, available randomized controlled trial evidence does not support current dietary fat guidelines.

Don't just sit there!

In the United States, people spend a lot of time sitting in front of the television, computer, and desk or using handheld devices. Break up your day by moving more and doing a normal aerobic activity that makes you sweat and breathe faster.

Get 2½ to 5 hours of moderate or vigorous-intensity physical activity each week. Go for a run, brisk walk or hike, play tennis, soccer, basketball, or hula hoop. Choose what you enjoy the most! By doing 10 minutes of physical activity at one time, several times throughout the day and the week, you will reach your goal for the total amount of physical activity you should do.

Strengthen your muscles at least twice a week. Do push-ups, pull-ups, lift weights, do heavy gardening, or work out with rubber resistance bands.

The Most Pressing Myths About Weight Loss

Food is asource that living beings from birth consume because the body needs nutrients to stay active. However, most people do not eat only when hungry, and other circumstances determine their intake.

Nutrition takes different concepts that are part of common knowledge. However, their meanings tend to be wider, making it necessary to delve into them. First, we have to clarify that "nutrition" is the set of processes through which nutrients are consumed, digested, absorbed, and used. Although it is sometimes used as a synonym for "food," this concept is much broader.

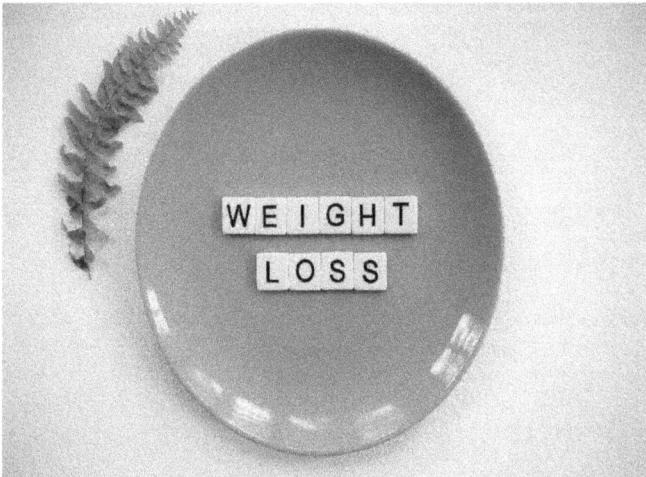

Through nutrition, your body can receive the energy and raw material that allows it to perform all its functions, such as forming tissues, renewing cells, performing physical activities, fighting an infection, among many others; that is why nutritionists design nutritional plans to starting from the requirements of each person.

Nutrition satisfies not only biological needs but also intellectual, emotional, aesthetic, and socio-cultural needs. For this reason, we will delve into the most common myths and truths within the field of nutrition. Join me!

Myth # 1: Diets are for weight loss.

Many people are scared by the word "diet" since the first thing that comes to mind is a restrictive food plan that allows them to reduce their weight or treat disease; however, in nutrition, this term is used to refer to the set of foods that anyone consumes during the day.

Fact: Everyone has a diet, but not necessarily for special or therapeutic purposes.

In case a person needs a special diet, we will specify the need in their plan, for example: "low-calorie diets" that are used to lose weight or "low-sugar diets" that are for patients with diabetes.

The food can be defined as any tissue, organ, or secretion from organisms of plant or animal origin. Some of their qualities are: they contain nutrients that the body can use, their consumption should not be harmful to health and vary depending on each culture. When considering the consumption of food to lose weight, ensure that the following characteristics are present:

BIOAVAILABILITY

That the nutrients can be digested and absorbed in your digestive system since it is useless to eat something that your body cannot use.

SAFETY

It refers to the quality standards that ensure that the product is free of dangers that can harm your body.

ACCESSIBILITY

That you can easily acquire it, check the availability in the market and the sale price.

SENSORY ATTRACTIVE

That it is pleasing to the senses; your sensory preferences are learned through repetitive exposure to certain flavors, textures, and aromas. Besides, each culinary style accentuates certain characteristics.

CULTURAL APPROVAL

Depending on the cultural group you are in, you get used to eating a certain food type. Eating habits depend on circumstances such as available food, collective experience, and economic capabilities.

Now that you know that diets refer to any type of food that people eat in their day-to-day life and know how to choose good food, let's get to know the following myths!

Myth # 2: To lose weight, you have to eat many meals a day

This is one of the myths that became very popular recently; one of the main reasons is that many people dedicated to sport had this custom. So that you understand it better, let us know the following case.

The Michael Phelps Diet

Even if you are not a sports fan, this name may sound familiar to you; Michael Phelps is a famous swimmer who holds the record for being the athlete with the most gold medals in all of the Olympics' history. He has training and consistency in his routine. Michael says that he swims for periods of 5-6 hours a day, six times a week;

Although Michael is the sample of someone who consumes several meals to speed up his metabolism and have enough energy, the eating plan is unique, individual, and according to each person's energy needs.

Reality: The energy requirements of each individual are different from those of other people and depend on factors such as:

1. Age

In each stage of growth, your need is greater, and it decreases as your age increases.

2. Sex

Generally, if you are a woman, you require between 5 and 10% fewer calories than a man.

3. Height

The higher the height, the requirement increases.

4. Physical activity

If you do intense physical activity, your energy consumption will be higher, so you will probably need more meals.

5. Health status

Your energy requirements change with different conditions, for example, if you are pregnant or if you have an infection or fever.

Don't be fooled! The best thing you can do to know the number of meals you need per day and the number of nutrients you should include is consulting a professional nutritionist. Let's go!

Myth # 3: Low-carb diets are best for weight loss

Carbohydrates, commonly known as carbohydrates, are the main source of energy in your diet. Proof of this is the first thing you think of when you are hungry since you prefer to eat a sandwich, cookies, sweet bread, tortillas, rice, pasta, etc. This happens because your body knows that you need energy.

It is likely that at some point, you have heard that to lose weight, you need to eliminate bread, tortillas, pasta, sugars, and all flours. This is not true! All food groups are important in our diet. If you want to know the necessary amounts in your case, you must inform yourself and learn from the experts.

There are several types of carbohydrates with variable functions and effects. If you want to include them in your diet healthy, you must know the amount you should eat depending on your energy needs.

Reality: Carbohydrates are the main source of energy for your cells and all your tissues. This force helps you run, breathe, make your heart work, think, and all your body activities every day.

Some other myths and truths have to do with weight reduction and the restrictions of certain foods and meals. These often damage health since they deprive the body of an important source of nutrients.

Myth # 4: If I skip meals, I will lose weight.

This myth is highly detrimental to health, so let's dive a little deeper into this aspect.

After eating, your liver glucose stores last for about 2 hours. When this energy source is depleted, your body uses the fat stores. Because this warehouse can last for weeks or months depending on your size, it seems like it pays to starve for hours; However, after 6 hours, your body changes its energy source again and looks for another way to obtain it.

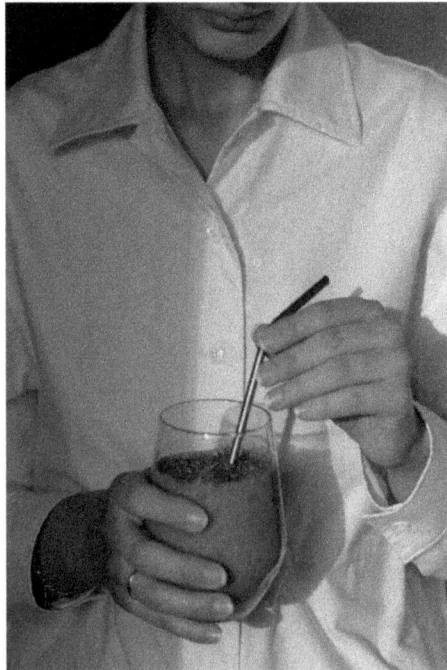

This is how it begins to take energy from proteins. This process is known as gluconeogenesis. This consumption method is not recommended since the main source of protein in the body is muscle mass, and this is not a reserve but a fabric with multiple functions. As a result, you will not only lose muscle mass, but you will also feel weak and accumulate more fat.

Reality: A balanced diet that considers the different nutritional needs during the day will allow you to lose weight.

It is very common that in magazines or the media, we hear about "miracle" diets suitable for all audiences. This belief has led us to think that it is unnecessary to consider aspects such as sex and age. This is what the following myth is about.

Myth # 5: Age is not a determining factor in diets.

Although age does not matter when designing a meal plan, an adult needs a different plan if it comes to losing weight or any other nutritional requirement.

To understand it better, let's look at how the total energy expenditure is managed:

- From 50 to 70% is occupied by the basal metabolism (cells). This percentage varies depending on the age, gender, and body weight of each person.

- From 6 to 10% is used to absorb nutrients from food.

- Finally, between 20 to 30% is occupied by physical activity, modified depending on habits and lifestyle.

Reality: From the analysis of age, gender, height, and the percentages of energy that each person requires, we can design a correct eating plan that allows you to lose weight if that is your goal.

The World Health Organization (WHO) recommends doing physical activity for 60 minutes, seven days a week. According to ENSANUT MC 2016, only 17.2% of people between 10 and 14 years old meet this recommendation; However, 77% of them spend more than two hours a day in front of the screen, on the other hand, 60% of adolescents between the ages of 15 and 19 consider that they are acting according to these criteria. Only 14.4% of adults meet this recommendation.

Are you within the 14.4% who are physically active or within the 85.6% who are inactive? Evaluate it, get to work, and get active!

Remember that your health is the most important thing. I hope that these myths about diet and their truths help you know how to stay in good condition. In case you need to lose weight, the best diet is the one that takes care of your health, don't forget it.

General Myths about Food

Myth: Eating meat is bad for my health and makes it harder for me to lose weight.

Truth: Eating small amounts of lean (low-fat) meat can be part of a healthy weight-loss plan. While it is true that chicken, fish, pork, and red meat contain some cholesterol and saturated fat, they also contain healthy nutrients like iron, protein, and zinc.

Tip: Select cuts of meat that are lower in fat and trim off any fat you see. Lean cuts of meat include chicken breast, pork loin, beef round steak, and extra-lean ground beef ("extra lean ground beef"). You should also look at your portion sizes. Try to eat your meat or chicken in 3-ounce (about 8.5 grams) or less.

Myth: Milk and milk products make me fat and unhealthy.

Truth: Fat-free or low-fat cheese, milk, and yogurt are just as nutritious as whole milk products, but they are lower in fat and calories. Milk products, also known as dairy products, have protein used to increase muscle mass and help the organs function well. They also have calcium that helps strengthen bones. Most milks and some yogurts are fortified with vitamin D, which helps the body use calcium. Most people who live in the United States do not get enough calcium, and vitamin D. Milk products are an easy way to get more of these nutrients.

Tip: According to government guidelines, you should aim for 3 cups a day of fat-free or low-fat milk or its equivalent in milk products. This can include vitamin-fortified soy-based drinks. If you cannot digest lactose (the type of sugar found in milk products), choose milk products lactose-free or low in lactose. You can also choose other foods and beverages that contain calcium and vitamin D, such as:

- Calcium: canned salmon, dark green leafy vegetables like collard greens or kale, and soy-based drinks or tofu made with calcium sulfate.
- Vitamin D: cereals or soy-based drinks.

Myth: Going vegetarian will help me lose weight and be healthier.

Truth: Studies show that people who follow a vegetarian meal plan generally consume fewer calories and fat than people who are not vegetarians. Some studies have also found that vegetarian-style eating is associated with a lower level of obesity, blood pressure, and heart disease risk. Vegetarians also have less body fat than non-vegetarians. However, both vegetarians and non-vegetarians can choose not-so-healthy foods that can affect their weight by causing them to gain. For example, they may eat large amounts of high fat and calories and with little nutritional value.

The types of vegetarian diets in the United States can vary greatly. Some people do not eat any animal product, while others consume milk and eggs along with plant foods. Some eat a vegetarian plan primarily but include small amounts of meat, seafood, chicken, or turkey.

Tip: If you decide to follow a vegetarian eating plan, be sure to get the nutrients that you normally get from animal products such as cheese, eggs, meat, and milk. In the table below, you will find a list of nutrients that may be missing from a vegetarian diet with some foods and drinks that may help you meet your needs for those nutrients.

The Core Principles of Nutrition

As the years go by, you begin to make your own decisions about many important things to you. You choose what to wear, what kind of music you like, and what friends you want to hang out with. Are you also ready to take charge of the decisions that affect your health?

This brochure highlights many things you can do to be healthier. Here you will find five important sections:

1. **Knowing how your body works** to explain how your body uses food and how physical activity and other tasks help the body "burn" the food you have eaten.

2. **Recharge your batteries with a healthy diet** that includes tips to help you eat healthier.

3. Get **Moving With Fun Activities** gives you some ideas to stay physically active and have fun at the same time.

4. **Stay Motivated and Keep** Going Share some ideas that help ease the transition to healthy habits and stick with them for a long time.

5. **Make It Work** is a practical tear-off sheet that can help you plan healthy meals and physical activities that fit your busy life.

You can also read the boxes titled "Did you know...?" to learn interesting facts about your health. Other helpful tips and entertaining ideas also appear throughout this page. You can flip through the brochure before you start reading it to give you an idea of what you will find.

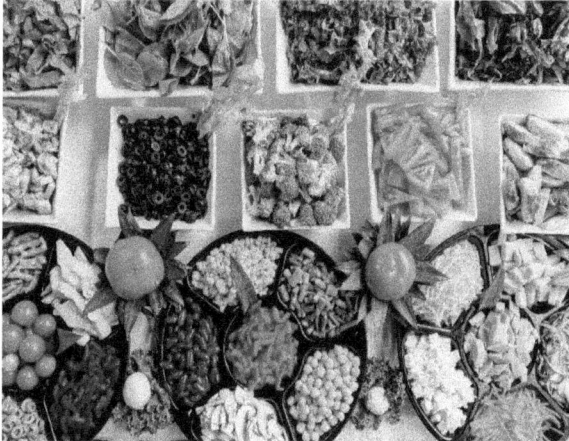

Know how your body works

Don't do it because "you're supposed to." Do it to take charge of your health!

Think of food as the energy that helps charge your batteries for the day. Throughout the day, you use the energy in those batteries to think and move, so you need to eat regularly to maintain this energy level. This is called "energy balancing" because you need to balance food (the energy you consume) with activity (the energy you burn).

How much energy does your body need?

You may have already heard about **calories**, which measure the amount of energy in a given food. There is no "right" number of calories that works for every person. The number of calories you need depends on whether you are a girl or a boy. It depends on your age and how active you are (which can vary from day to day).

Should you go on a diet?

Dieting may not be the sensible thing to do. Many teens try to lose weight by eating too little, not eating, skipping meals, and cutting out food groups entirely, such as carbohydrates or "carbs." These methods can bypass important foods your body needs. Unhealthy diets can cause you togain more weight because they often lead to a cycle where you eat too little and then eat too much. After all, you're hungry.

Other weight-loss tactics such as smoking, making yourself vomit, or using diet pills or laxatives (medicines that help people have a bowel movement) can also lead to health problems.

Eating healthy and being physically active can help you...

- Do better in school.
- Have friends who share your interests in dance, sports, and other activities.
- Tone and strengthen muscles.
- Improve your mood.

Recharge your batteries with a healthy diet

Healthy eating includes taking control of the amount and type of foods you eat. This section has information that will help you.

- Control your food portions.
- Charge your batteries with high-energy foods.
- Avoid pizza, sweets, and fast foods.
- Stay energized all day.

Control your food portions.

A serving is the amount of one of the foods consumed at a given time. Many people eat larger portions than they need, especially when eating out. Ready-to-go meals (from a restaurant, grocery store, or school event) can have portions even larger than you need.

When eating at home ...

- Take a serving out of the package and serve it on a plate instead of eating it straight out of a box or bag. "What do all those numbers mean?" See the section below for an explanation of where to find serving sizes.

- Avoid eating while watching television or while you are busy doing other activities. It's easy to lose track of how much you eat while doing other things.

- Eat slowly, so your brain gets the message that your stomach is full. Your brain needs about twenty minutes before receiving the message.

- Think twice before serving yourself again. Are you still hungry, or are you just helping yourself to more because the food tastes good?

- Try not to snack after dinner.

When eating out ...

- Ask for something small. Try eating half a serving or a healthy snack, like hummus (chickpea spread) with whole wheat pita bread or grilled chicken. If you order a large meal, take half home, or share it with someone else at the table.

- Limit the amount of "fast food" you eat. When shopping for "fast food," say "no thanks" to extra-large or special-size options, such as specials sold with French fries and sodas.

Did you know?

Just one oversized "fast food" plate can have more calories than you should eat a whole day. And when people are served more food, they eat more — even when they don't need it. This can result in weight gain.

Recharge your batteries with high-energy foods.

Healthy eating is not just about the amount of food you eat. You need to make sure that you eat the type of food that your body needs. Try to eat foods that include fruits, vegetables, whole grains, low-fat protein, and dairy products. Here's more information, and at the end of this guide, you can also see the tear-off sheet for planning meals.

Fruits and vegetables

Serve half the plate with fruits and vegetables. Dark green, red, and orange vegetables, in particular, have high levels of the kinds of nutrients you need, such as vitamin C, calcium, and fiber. Nutrients — such as vitamins, minerals, and dietary fiber — nourish the body, giving it what it needs to be healthy. Adding spinach or lettuce and tomato to your sandwich is an easy way to include vegetables in your meal.

Grain

Choose to eat whole grains, such as whole-wheat bread or tortillas, brown rice, oatmeal, and multigrain enchiladas.

Protein

Fuel up on lean meats like turkey on a sandwich or chicken, seafood, eggs, beans, unsalted nuts, tofu, and other protein-rich foods.

Dairy foods

Build strong bones with fat-free or low-fat dairy products. If your body can't digest lactose (the sugar in milk that causes stomach pain in some people), opt for soy milk or rice milk and low-fat yogurt.

Did you know?

Many teens don't get enough of their four nutrients:

- **Calcium** builds strong bones and teeth.
- **Vitamin D** supports bone health.
- **Potassium** helps lower blood pressure.
- **Dietary fiber** can improve the digestion of food and help you feel full.
- **Protein** helps you grow strong and gives you energy.
- **Iron** supports your development.

Put a limit on pizzas, desserts, "fast foods," and sodas.

You don't have to stop eating all of these things, but eating them in smaller amounts can help you maintain a healthy weight. Pizza, desserts, "fast food," and soda contain added sugar, solid fats, and sodium. A healthy eating plan is low in these additives.

Added sugar

Many foods, especially fruits, are naturally sweet. Other foods, such as cookies, cakes (or cakes), and mini chocolate cakes, have added sugar to taste better. Sugar adds calories but not nutrients such as vitamins that help your body grow and function well.

Maintain a healthy weight

- Try to eat fewer foods like cookies and candy. If you eat desserts, try low-fat frozen yogurt.
- Avoid adding sugar to your meals and sodas.
- Drink water, low-fat or fat-free milk, and avoid beverages that are high in sugar. Sodas, energy sodas, and juices contribute a large part of the added sugar to our diet.

Solid fats

Fat is important. It helps your body grow and develop. It is a source of energy. And it keeps your skin and hair healthy. But some fats are better than others.

Solid fats are solid at room temperatures, such as butter, stick margarine, shortening, and lard. These often contain saturated fat and trans fat, which are high in calories and not healthy for your heart. Try to avoid foods like cakes, cookies, pizza, and potato chips, which often contain a lot of solid fat.

Did you know?

Not all fats are unhealthy! Some fats are healthy — as long as you don't eat them in large amounts. Try to eat a moderate amount of the following foods that have healthier fats:

- Olive, canola, safflower, sunflower, and soybean oils
- Fish, such as tuna, salmon, and trout

Sodium

Your body needs a small amount of sodium (which is mainly found in salt). But eating too much sodium can raise your blood pressure, which is unhealthy for your heart and your body in general.

Processed foods, those that come canned, frozen, or packaged, often contain a lot of sodium. Fresh foods are sodium-free, but they often cost more. If you can afford the expense, eat fresh food, and make your low-salt meals. If you eat packaged meals, look at the amount of sodium listed on the Nutrition Facts label. (See the section titled "What do all these numbers mean?" Wash canned vegetables to remove excess salt.

Try to eat less than 2,300 mg of sodium a day. This amount is equivalent to one teaspoon and includes salt that already comes in prepared foods and the salt you add when you cook or serve food.

Your doctor knows more about your special needs; so don't hesitate to ask how much sodium you should eat.

What do all these numbers mean?

When you read a food label, pay special attention to:

The serving size. Look at the amount of food in one serving. Do you eat more or less than that? The line that says "servings per container" tells you the number of servings in that food package.

Calories and other nutrients. Remember that the number of calories and other nutrients listed on the label is only one serving. Food packages often contain more than one serving.

Percent Daily Value (DV). See how much of the recommended daily amount of a nutrient (Percent Daily Value) (% DV) is in a serving of food. In most cases, 5% DV or less is considered a low value, and 20% DV or more is considered a high value. For example, this label shows that food has 15% of the calcium you need to eat in a day. We can consider that this food has a high level of calcium. It should also be noted that it also has a high sodium level (28%).

Eat healthy snacks

- Fresh apples, strawberries, or grapes
- A small bag of carrots
- Low-fat or fat-free yogurt
- Low-fat string cheese
- Peanut butter on whole-grain crackers

Did you know?

Canteens who eat breakfast do better in school and sports — and have a healthier weight?

Stay energized all day

Skipping meals can lead to weight gain. Follow these tips to maintain a healthy weight:

- **Have breakfast every day.** This makes your body go. You can have something in the way, such as a piece of fruit and a slice of whole-wheat bread.
- **Pack your food or lunch on the days you have to go to school**. If you pack your food or lunch, you can control the portions and ensure that your food is healthy.
- **Eat healthy snacks and try not to skip meals.** Read the ideas in the "Eat healthy snacks" paragraph.
- **Dinner with your family.** When you eat dinner with your family, you are more likely to eat a healthy meal and can take the time to catch up with the rest of the family.
- **Participate in grocery shopping and meal planning at home.** By participating, you can make sure your meals are healthy and taste good.

Eat healthy without spending too much money

Try these tips:

- Help your parents buy inexpensive generic brand products, such as whole-grain bread, pasta, and other healthy items.
- Eat at home when possible.
- Pack a healthy meal or lunch and snacks, so you don't have to spend money on food when you go out.
- Take a bottle of water with you. Fill it in a source of water when necessary.

Moving on

Being physically active can help you control your weight, increase your flexibility and balance. You don't have to have boring exercise routines. You can be active during your daily activities, such as taking the stairs instead of taking the elevator or escalator. Or you can get around doing fun activities like dancing or playing sports.

This section can help you:

- Be active every day.
- Go outdoors.
- Have fun with your friends.
- Stay active if they are indoors too.

Be active every day

Physical activity should be part of your daily life, whether it's playing sports, having physical education classes or other exercise classes, or even walking or cycling from place to place. You should be physically active for 60 minutes every day, but you don't have to do it all at once!

Did you know?

Doing physical activity is supposed to be simple and fun. Here's a way to get 60 minutes of activity:

+ 10 minutes - walk or bike to a friend's house

+ 30 minutes - throw the ball into the basket

+ 20 minutes - dance

60 minutes of activity

Be active with your friends and family

Being active can be more fun with friends or family members. You may also find that you can make new friends when you join active clubs or participate in community activities. Together with your family or friends, teach each other games or activities and keep things interesting by choosing a different activity every day, for example:

- playing soccer, basketball, volleyball, tennis, or another favorite sport
- going for a walk or bike ride with a family member or friend

You could even sign up with your friends to have fun, to go to live events like fundraisers, hikes, fun runs, or treasure hunts.

What if I don't have money to get sports equipment?

You don't need money or equipment to stay active. You can dance or use the free facilities offered by your community to do your daily 60-minute physical activities. If you want to play a sport or game that requires equipment, ask your neighbors or friends at school if they can loan you equipment or if they can share the sporting goods you need with you.

It goes out into the open air.

Being active outdoors gives you the daily activity you need, and sunlight helps improve your vitamin D levels. Many teens spend a lot of time indoors watching television, surfing the internet, or playing video games. Let's call the time you spend doing these activities,"screentime." While these activities can relax you after a long day at school, spending too much time in front of the screen can lead to weight gain and health-related other problems. Instead, spending time outdoors can help you burn calories and improve your vitamin D level if the day is sunny.

Decrease the time in front of the screen:

- Record your favorite shows and watch them later. This will cut down on TV time because that way, you plan to watch specific shows instead of searching and switching from channel to channel.

- Replace the time you spend watching television and playing video games with physical activities. Get involved in activities at your school or in your community.

- Gradually decrease the time you spend using your phone, computer, or television.

- Set a time slot with your friends without texting each other, a period that allows you to be physically active together and agree not to text or reply to each other.

- Take breaks if you spend sitting in front of the computer. Go for a walk, clean your room, anything that gives your body movement.

- Turn off your mobile phone before going to sleep.

Choose activities that you like

Being physically active doesn't mean you have to be a gym member or play a team sport. Try some of the following ideas:

- Play basket.

- Ride a bike (wear a helmet).

- Run.

- Go skateboarding.

- Jump rope or use a hoop or hula hoop.

- Have a dance party with your friends?

- Play volleyball or flag football.

- Get moving with a video game that tracks your movements.

Be careful with the media.

Ads, TV shows, the Internet, and other media can affect how you choose to eat and spend your time. Many advertisements try to convince you to eat high-fat foods and sweetened sodas. Others may try to sell you products, like video games. Watch out for some of these tricks that commercials use to pressure you:

- An ad may show a group of young people eating a meal or using a product to make you think that all young people do the same or should do the same. The ad may use words such as "All youth need ..." or "All youth are ..."

- Advertisers sometimes show famous players using or recommending a product because they think you will want to buy products that your favorite stars wear.

- Commercials often use cartoons to make it seem like fun and good food or activity for young people.

Stay active indoors too.

When there are cold days or when it rains, spending time in front of the screen is not the only option. Find ways to be active indoors:

- Play indoor sports or active games in your building, at home, or a local recreation center.

- Dance to your favorite music alone or with friends.

- If you have a video game system, choose active dance and sports games that follow your movements.

Take your time

- **Make changes slowly.** Don't expect to change your eating or activity habits from one day to the next. Changing too many things too quickly can hurt your chances of success.

- **Find ways to make your eating and physical activity habits healthier.** Keep a food and activity diary for about four to five days and write down everything you eat, the activities you do, and your emotions. Check the journal to get an idea of your habits. Do you skip breakfast? Are you physically active most days of the week? Do you eat when you are stressed? You can keep a journal in a notebook, on a piece of paper, or your computer.

- **Know what is affecting you.** Do you have snacks at home that are too tempting? Does your cafeteria food have too much fat and added sugar? Do you find it difficult not to be able to resist drinking several sweetened sodas a day because your friends drink them?

- **Set some realistic goals for yourself.** First of all, try to replace some sodas you drink (for example, sodas, some juices, and energy drinks) with unsweetened beverages. Once you drink less soda, try eliminating all soda. Then set some more goals, like drinking low-fat or skim milk, eating more fruit, or being more physically active every day.

- **Get a friend from school or someone at home to support you in your new habits.** Ask a friend or family member to help you make these changes and stick with new habits.

- **Convince yourself that you can do it!** Use the information in this booklet and the resources in the next section to help you. Stay positive and focused, always remembering why you want to be healthier - to look, feel, and move better. Accept the setbacks that may arise; If you don't meet one of your daily eating or physical activity goals, don't give up. Just try the next day again.

You can achieve it!

Changing your habits is difficult. Developing new habits takes time. Use the tips below, as well as the tear-off tip sheet and checklist at the end of this guide, to stay motivated and meet your goals.

Make it work!

Being healthy seems like it takes a lot of work, right? It doesn't have to be that way. Use this tear-off sheet to help you plan your healthy meals and incorporate healthy habits into your day. Post this list on your snack or school locker to serve as a practical reminder.

Examples of meals

Breakfast: a cup of low-sugar whole-grain cereal with low-fat milk and topped with a sliced banana

Meal or lunch: a turkey sandwich with cheese, dark leaf lettuce, tomato, and red bell peppers on whole wheat bread

Dinner: grilled chicken with salad

Make healthy habits a part of your day.

Healthy habits and being active can be difficult because you spend so much of your day at school and eat meals prepared by other people. Be a Champion of Health, participating more in your meals and school activities. Here is a list to help you incorporate healthy habits into your daily life.

BE A HEALTH CHAMPION!

- Every night, prepare and pack your food or lunch and snacks for the next day.

- Go to bed at the same time every night to recharge your mind and body. At bedtime, be sure to turn off your cell phone, TV, and other gadgets.

- Eat breakfast.

- Walk or bike to school if you live nearby and can do it safely.

- Drink water all day. Avoid sodas and other high-calorie drinks.

- Between classes, stand up and walk around, even if the next class is in the same room.

- If your school allows recess, be sure to walk, jump rope, or play an active game with your friends.

- Be active during your physical education class.

- At lunch or lunch, eat what you packed. If you have money to eat or lunch, spend it on healthy options. Avoid soda, potato chips, and candy from vending machines.

- Get active after school hours by joining a sports team or dance group. Clean your room or take part in an impromptu soccer or softball game.

- Participate in the food options of your house. Help prepare dinner and eat with your family.

- Save the time you spend in front of the screen after your activities and limit that time to less than two hours a day.

Do you have doubts about how to eat a healthy diet? I understand you, for a long time I did not know what to eat, and I was very confused if what I chose was good for me or not.

In this section, I will talk about healthy eating principles that do not go out of style because it is not about a diet but about giving your body what it needs to be healthy and full of energy.

Unfortunately, the information on healthy eating that we can find on the internet is very contradictory. In one place, you find it as something great for your health. In another place, they put it as the worst thing you could eat.

What diet is the best?

What is the correct diet? Paleo Diet, Vegetarian, Vegan, Raw-Vegan, Macrobiotic Diet, Ketogenic Diet, Mediterranean Diet… There are hundreds of diets and eating styles.

The truth is that we cannot declare a winning diet.Each of them has benefits and also has certain consequences when it is not handled properly.

Also, there is a fundamental principle that health coaches call: **BIO-INDIVIDUALITY**.

This means that each person is different and has needs that are unlike anyone else's. The diet that could be perfect for that person cannot favor another person.

Therefore, no diet suits everyone.

A healthy diet is like a pair of shoes. For them to be comfortable and you can walk long distances with them, they need to be tailor-made for you.

Your shoes will surely not fit your mother or friends because they have their size and shape characteristics in their feet.

Now that you know that there is no "perfect diet" for everyone, the question is, what should I eat to have a healthy diet?

Healthy eating is not about practicing strict philosophies, staying unrealistically slim, or depriving yourself of the foods you love.

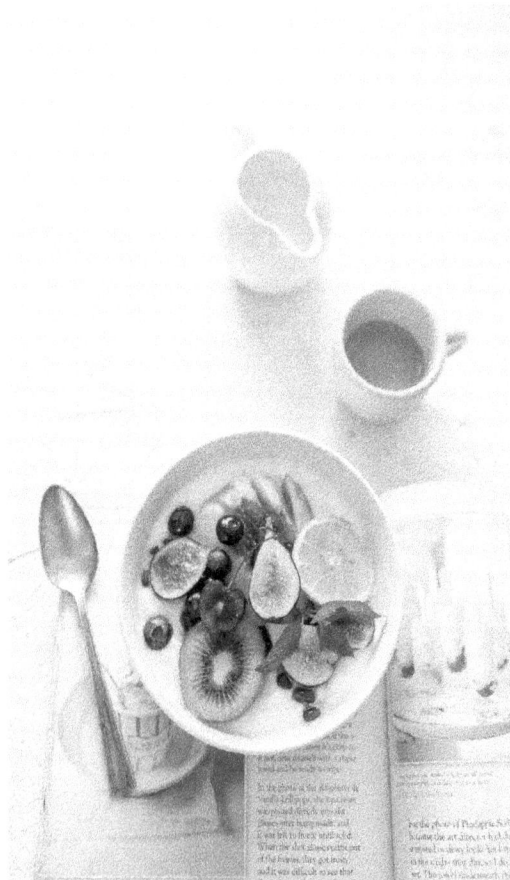

Instead, it's about eating smart to feel great, have high energy, and stay healthy for the long haul. All of this can be achieved by learning the basic principles of healthy eating and adjusting them to your life as much as possible.

Eating healthy starts with eating smart. It's about what we eat and also how we eat it.

With our choices, we can reduce the risk of heart disease, cancer, and diabetes, as well as defend ourselves against depression. In addition, **healthy habits** can make us feel full of energy, improve our memory, and stabilize our mood.

With each new food you try, you can expand the range of foods you eat. That's great to help you differentiate between what you like, what your body likes, and what makes you happy.

Learning to eat well and feel happy is one of the most important things in our life because that directly influences the quality we are going to live the rest of our existence.

How to Get Started?

1. Small constant changes

To be successful, let's think about small steps or changes rather than big sacrifices. Instead of obsessing over calories or food portions, let's think of our diet as full of color, variety, and freshness.

Your food is not your enemy, but the life force you need to feel full of energy and to make your cells work at their best.

Trying to change our diet radically is unrealistic and frustrates us if we don't achieve our goals quickly. Let's make small changes to healthy eating, like adding a salad filled with different colors each day, topped with olive oil instead of bottled dressings.

Once those changes have become a habit, you can try new changes that are more challenging over time.

The goal is not to be perfect or exaggerated. To be healthy and fit, we do not need to go on a strict diet. Nor is it necessary to eliminate our favorite foods forever to achieve a healthy diet.

All the foods that we know that do not benefit us have a healthy version that you could prepare at home do not benefit us in the long run. Therefore, the goal is to feel good, have a healthy weight, prevent illness, and enjoy food wisely and that this is sustainable in the long term.

We also have to consider that we don't just need food to flourish. We also need to nourish ourselves with good exercise, natural water, and harmonious relationships, especially with ourselves.

2. Moderation is the key to healthy eating

Restrictive diets (eliminate one or more food groups) don't work in the long run, or they can be dangerous.

Especially if they focus on eliminating one or more food groups from our diet.

We all need all three macronutrients to function properly: proteins, carbohydrates, and fats, as well as fiber, vitamins, minerals, and water. None of this can be absent because our bodies would get sick.

For a healthy diet, I recommend ZERO PROHIBITIONS.

When we ban certain foods during a diet, we crave more. By "falling" into temptation, we believe that we have failed, making us feel very unmotivated.

If you like to eat unhealthy or very sweet foods, start by reducing your portions and eating them less often.

You will see that each time you will remember less of them, or the craving will decrease. This will especially be true when you start substituting these foods for real, nutritious food.

Think in smaller portions. Especially when you eat in restaurants, the portions they serve you are huge. They have grown in the last few years and from normal size have gone to EXTRA JUMBO.

When you eat out, you can share those huge dishes with your companions, and if you are already feeling satisfied, you can order to take the food or simply leave it on the plate.

Especially meats come in exaggerated sizes. A suitable portion should be the size of a deck of cards or cards.

3. It's not what you eat, but how you eat it

Eating healthy goes beyond food. It is about what we think about it.

Question your behavior. Is it about filling your belly or being well nourished?

Is it a matter of sharing with others or eating alone and in a hurry? Do you enjoy the flavors, smells, textures, and combinations of your food?

Do you eat with a variety, or do you go for monotonous options? Do you listen to your body when you are hungry, thirsty, or satisfied?

Do you feel the difference between hunger and thirst? Do you give importance to breakfast and healthy snacks?

Those answers will help you assess whether you need to change your eating habits. Those small adjustments will help you eat more mindfully and enjoy your food more than viewing it as an enemy.

4. Color is very important

Fruits and vegetables are the basic points of a good diet. They are low in calories and high in nutrients like vitamins, minerals, antioxidants, and fiber. They must be present in all our meals, including snacks.

When you eat a plant-based diet, it is difficult to be overweight for two reasons.

1. The first is because whole fruits (not juiced) and vegetables are high in fiber.

Fiber is the indigestible part of food that expands in your stomach and intestines and gives you a malaise feeling. When you are satisfied, there is not much room for unhealthy food.

2. The second reason is that especially vegetables contain very few calories. Therefore, they help you eat until you feel satisfied, without eating very caloric foods that turn into fat in the **waist and hips**.

They have recommended that we eat a minimum of 5 servings of fruits and vegetables a day, to start is fine. Today, we know that **consuming between 7 and 10 servings** helps prevent and treat problems such as cancer, heart disease, arthritis, diabetes, and obesity.

If you think that ten servings could be a lot, try different ways to prepare your vegetables. For example, it is easy to eat 3 or 4 servings in a **smoothie**.

5. Choose whole grains

Healthy carbohydrate sources are whole grains. I'm not talking **about boxed breakfast cereals** or white bread. I am referring to whole-grain bread, cookies, and pasta made with corn, barley, brown rice, whole oats, rye, quinoa, beans, lentils, and other legumes, fruits, and vegetables.

Healthy carbohydrates are absorbed slowly, so they keep your energy levels constant and your feeling of being full for longer.

Unhealthy carbohydrates are those such as white flour, refined sugar, and its derivatives. These do not contain fiber or other nutrients.

This causes them to be absorbed quickly and cause a sudden rise in blood sugar and then fall also abruptly. This makes you hungry or craving after eating or eventually leads to insulin resistance or diabetes.

Tip: Avoid bread, pasta, and cereals that are not whole grains by reading the label and looking for more than 2 grams of fiber per serving. And eat them in moderation.

6. Eat healthy fats

Fats are needed to nourish our brain, heart, and all cells. They are also responsible for keeping skin, hair, and nails healthy.

There is no healthy diet without fat. But next the importance of choosing good sources of fat.

The good fats to INCREASE are:

Monounsaturated fats: olive oil, avocado, walnuts, and other seeds like almonds, sesame, and pumpkin.

Polyunsaturated fats (including omega 3): Fish oils such as salmon, anchovies, sardines, and tuna. Also, oils such as linseed oil.

The fats to REDUCE are:

Saturated fats: Of animal origins like the fat of meats and whole dairy products. Butter, lard, and fatty cheeses.

The fats to be ELIMINATED:

Trans fats: Found in margarine, cookies, candy, snacks, fried foods, tamales, pastries, and other industrial foods that contain "partially hydrogenated oils" or burnt oils.

7. Choose high-quality protein

Protein is made up of 20 different building blocks called amino acids. They serve to build tissues and repair our bodies. Also, to form enzymes and hormones essential for life.

A low-protein diet can slow children's growth, reduce muscle mass, lower our immune system, weaken the heart, and cause respiratory problems at any age.

Proteins are not only found in meats. We can find them in beans, lentils, other legumes, walnuts, almonds, and other seeds, besides soy foods such as tofu, soy milk and tempeh, hemp seeds, quinoa, algae, and spirulina.

The amounts of protein we eat are generally larger than we need. Try that on your plate. The size of the meat is not larger than the portion of vegetables.

Another way to measure the amount of meat is that it is no larger than the size of the palm of your hand.

If you have any questions about your protein intake or are vegan or vegetarian, consult a plant-based diet specialist. It will help you determine your protein requirements and show you which sources are best suited for you.

Remember that it is possible to have a healthy vegan diet, but quality information is required to avoid putting your body in a risky and unhealthy situation.

8. Add calcium to your diet

It is one of the most important nutrients for a healthy diet. We need 1000 mg of calcium a day. It is advisable to consume low-fat dairies such as cheese or yogurt and other foods rich in calcium. If you are vegan, there are many sources of calcium in green leafy vegetables and seeds.

Foods high in calcium are milk, yogurt, and cheese. Vegetables with calcium are dark green, as are squash, peas, Brussels sprouts, and mushrooms. Beans of any kind also contain calcium and sesame seeds.

9. Avoid processed foods

If your diet contains fruits, vegetables, whole grains, lean proteins, and good fats, you will find that you can automatically reduce the amount of **junk food**.

It is like a scale, and more than removing food, it is about including all the foods mentioned above.

Even if you avoid sweets, desserts very high in sugar, and unhealthy snacks, you should know that sugar is often "hidden" in processed foods.

Bread, canned goods, pasta sauces, margarine, mashed potatoes, frozen food, fast food, dressings, ketchup, and beverages are full of unhealthy sugars.

Avoid sugary drinks. One soda contains ten teaspoons of sugar. This is more than the recommendation for one day. It's too much.

Include naturally sweet foods like fruit, beets, carrots, bell peppers, or yellow corn to satisfy your sweet flavors' craving.

Remember that on the labels, we can find sugar with different names:

Cane sugar or maple syrup, corn syrup, honey or molasses, agave syrup, high fructose corn syrup, fruit concentrate, maltodextrin, dextrose, fructose, glucose, maltose, or sucrose.

Any of these names indicate that they are ingredients that are not good to consume frequently.

Try to limit your salt intake. In a healthy diet, we need 1,200 to 2,300 mg of sodium a day, the equivalent of one teaspoon of salt.

To achieve this, reduce packaged foods, prefer fresh vegetables and fruits instead of canned ones, and reduce salty snacks such as potatoes and peanuts. And please take the salt shaker off the table.

10. Drink more water

Water is what your body needs, not sodas or processed juices, teas, and coffee.

Most of our body is made up of water, and every day through urine, sweat, and digestion, we lose a lot of water.

That is the reason why I advise you to drink at least eight glasses of natural water. If you do a lot of sports or live in a very hot climate, you will need more water.

Thirst is often mistaken for hunger, so the next time you are about to fit your tooth into the chocolate cake, drink a glass or two of water and check if the feeling you mistook for hunger was not thirst.

By following these ten principles of healthy eating, you can be sure that you are developing healthy habits to stay healthy and fit in the long term.

Remember to take baby steps to build healthy eating until you feel more confident about making more drastic changes.

Step by step, you get to Rome.

Chapter 2: #MakeTheShift – Being Plant-Based

The advantages of a plant-based diet are wonderful. At the same time, we help the planet and animals. They are also easy to prepare, and it is a simple way to include our children in preparing meals.

A couple of weeks ago, I joined the **One Meal A Day** Challenge and announced it on Facebook since many people write to me to ask how they can implement a plant-based diet or how they can be vegan without dying in the attempt.

But before I tell you about this challenge, I want to tell you about One Meal A Day and the advantages of a plant-based diet, since many of us have awakened to the reality of our world, and no matter what the reason is. If you want a change in your life and that of your family, it is important to know that we are not alone on the journey and that together we are achieving a great change in our health and planet.

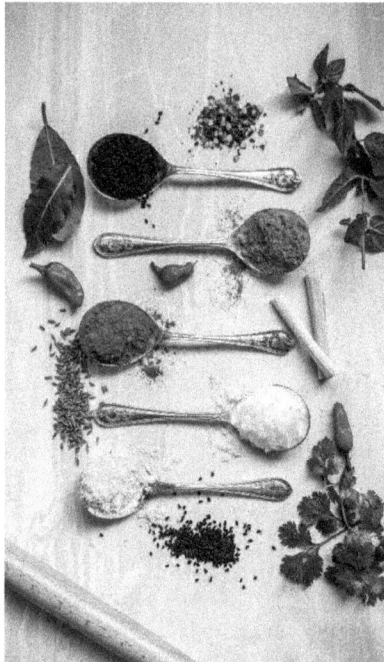

OMD is a campaign based on the upcoming book by Suzy Amis Cameron - She wants to advocate for people to go plant-based for just one meal a day. Your community is designed to support and inspire people to make an accessible change for their health and the future of the planet - one bite at a time.

When I learned about One Meal A Day at a California conference, I was fascinated by the support they provide for people to eat more plant-based foods. Still, I was more delighted that they are changing the food system to improve access to food options, healthy food across the country, including schools, a critical issue for our children's future.

Starting a plant-based (vegan) diet is very difficult for most people. Letting go of old habits; learning about what to eat and what not to eat is not easy.

Substituting healthy foods for meat and processed foods can sometimes put some off. These tips can help you make the change.

Understand that it is a process

Making any life changes, especially those related to food, is a process that does not happen overnight.

To make the transition easier and more enjoyable, have realistic expectations. You know yourself, and you can define how to beat old habits step by step and celebrate every time you reach a small goal.

Most people choose to follow a plant diet primarily for health. After they know more about healthy eating, they affirm the decision for other reasons.

To begin the change, define the reason why you are trying to change your diet. Then set specific, achievable milestones with a due date.

For example, some goals could be:

- **Eat a serving of vegetables at each meal starting in the first week.**
- **Learn to cook three new healthy meals per month.**

Put these lenses somewhere where you can see them often. This will remind you of your goals and why you are making the change. This will help you do them.

Add, do not subtract

One of the reasons many people give up on their goals is that they try to make too big changes too fast. If you have decided to eat a healthier diet, start small, and consider adding new foods instead of eating family meals. Do you like pasta? Substitute wheat pasta or brown rice with arugula and sun-dried tomatoes. Do you like to eat something sweet in the morning? Try a vanilla shake with frozen almond milk and banana, fresh spinach, and a hemp seed protein. Do you tend to have dinner every day? Start your meal with a colorful salad or a bowl of homemade vegetable soup, and you will be able to increase your vegetable intake while reducing the main course.

Small, simple, and manageable changes add up and bring in new good habits over time.

Learn to cook

One of the best things you can do for your health is to learn how to prepare meals at home. Only by cooking can you control the ingredients you cook with.

In many restaurants and processed foods, sodium is used in exaggerated amounts to flavor and preserve foods. When you cook, you can replace it with aromatic spices.

If you've never cooked before, start small to prepare simple dinners. Soups and curries are great for beginners because they are almost impossible to get off.

If you are already an experienced cook, decide to level up. Take on the challenge of preparing dishes with more ingredients from scratch.

Learn to:

- Cook your beans instead of using canned ones.
- Prepare a style of food that you are not as familiar with as vegetarian Indian food.

The more you cook, the more control you have over what you eat and your health.

Get inspired

If you are eating the same dishes every week or are beginning to lose the drive to make healthy changes, this is the time to seek inspiration.

Take a look at some new cookbooks, cooking magazines, online recipe sites like this one. Or visit a vegetarian or vegan restaurant in your city or a neighboring city.

Go shopping at a local farmers' market. Not only is it better for the planet to eat local and seasonal fruits and vegetables, but they are more affordable, healthier, and tastier.

Farmers' markets also allow you to explore new fruits and vegetables and discover recipe suggestions from the farmers themselves.

Seek support

It's always easier and more enjoyable to make the change with a friend or family member's support. Mutual help helps you make healthy changes.

Swap recipes and try new restaurants together. Having a "health buddy" can help you feel supported in your decision to eat healthily and stick with your purpose.

Don't stress

Food should be enjoyable, not stressful. If you find yourself worried or stressed about your progress (or perhaps a lack of progress), find out why you feel this way. Are you trying to make too many changes at once? Are you stuck and don't know how to proceed? Are you losing your momentum and the reason that led you to decide to change? Once you discover the cause of stress, it is much easier to find a way to manage it and make your transition to healthier eating more enjoyable.

Be kind to yourself

Now and then, we all crave less healthy foods. Don't feel guilty if an additional treat is allowed from time to time (a little chocolate here and there is not bad). However, if you find yourself continually eating dessert each night, then you should consider prioritizing your decision to eat healthier.

Obsessing over and punishing yourself for unhealthy eating will not inspire you to want to change - it will only make you feel guilty. Nobody likes to feel guilty, and it is certainly not fun to associate food with guilt. Be patient with yourself and know that no one has a perfect diet. However, making healthier choices will help you achieve a healthy and happy lifestyle.

Making Up Your Mind

Would you like to lose weight?

Would you like to feel better?

Would you like to improve, stabilize, or even get to reverse a chronic disease such as heart disease, high cholesterol, diabetes, or high blood pressure?

Would you like to take less medicine?

Would you be willing to try a diet different if it could improve your health?

If you answered "yes" to any of the above questions, a plant-based diet might be adequate for you. This brochure includes information to help you follow a low-fat diet consisting of unprocessed and plant-based natural foods.

My action plan

An action plan allows you to break down your goal of changing your diet to a plant-based diet into manageable parts. Havingan action plan supports your chances of success. Preparing your plan should include detailed steps and do the following questions:

• *What* will *you* do?

• *How much* will *you* do?

• *When* will you do it?

• *How many days* a week will you do it?

Example:

This week I'll have a salad *(what)* with 3 cups *(how much)* tomatoes, carrots, chickpeas and cucumber for dinner *(when)* on Monday, Wednesday and Friday *(how many days)*.

This week I:

_____ *(what)*

_____ *(how much)*

_____ *(when)*

_____ *(how many days)*

How important is it to you to change your diet?

0

1

2

3

4

5

6

7

8

9

10

0 = nothing important

10 = very important

Congratulations on taking such an important step for the benefit of yourhealth andwellness.

If it turns out that you can't eat a 100% vegetarian diet percent, try to follow it at 80 percent. Remember that any effort you make to consume more vegetables and fruits and less meat and animal products can improve your health.

Plant-based, vegetarian, and vegan food can be super healthy and energetic in any life cycle if it is done in a complete and varied way. Incorporating more real food into the daily diet. Adding fresh vegetables and fruits, seeds, whole grains, legumes, nuts, algae, superfoods such as maca, spirulina provide the body with quality food and all the necessary nutrients for proper functioning, purifying it, and recovering its self-healing capacity.

The key is to stop consuming so many packages, ultra-processed products with base ingredients such as wheat flour, corn, soy, sugar, fats, full of chemicals, flavorings, and colorings that do not nourish and generate addiction. Everything vegan is not synonymous with healthy. Many vegan foods fall into these groups when eaten in excesses, such as seitan, soybeans, commercial cookies, dressings, sodas, and others.

By basing the highest number of intakes on plants, you transform the diet into a more alkaline and physiological one, incorporating food-medicine among its many benefits:

- Plants are high in fiber, which provides satiety, controls glucose absorption avoiding blood glucose peaks, and stimulates proper evacuation.

- They have antioxidants, prevent premature aging, have anti-cancer, and neuroprotective anti-inflammatory effects.

- They have a high concentration of vitamins and minerals: consuming whole plants provides a good dose of vitamins and minerals, enzymatic cofactors of many metabolic reactions in the body, which stimulates the general biochemical functionality of the body, increases energy, and improves the state of spirit.

- They are purifying. They help eliminate toxins through our purifying organs, liver, kidney through urine, fecal matter, and sweat.

- They alkalize the body, which helps compensate for acidosis caused by excess consumption of meats or processed foods.

It is important to accompany the transition to a *plant-based* diet - vegan or vegetarian - with complete blood tests with a dose of vitamin B12 and homocysteine to evaluate the state of health and supplementation protocol since it is not covered with foods of plant origin. It is very normal that in cases of flexible vegetarians without nutritional control after a time has passed since the change of diet, the values are low, and symptoms appear.

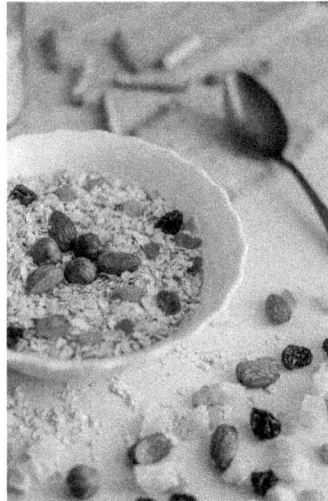

Where do you get proteins from?

It may be the most heard question when living this change in habits. When you stop consuming meats, eggs, and dairy, it is important to consider protein supplementation to cover all essential amino acids. In the plant kingdom, amino acids are distributed in different foods: cereals, legumes, seeds, algae, sprouts, nuts, mushrooms, nutritional yeast. By correctly supplementing them, we ensure the supply of proteins. That is why we always add some of these foods to the dishes. There are different ways to do it: you can add to a plate cereal with legumes, more fresh vegetables of different colors, activated seeds, and a complete meal rich in all the essential amino acids. Another way is to consume cereals or legumes with nuts, algae, seeds, sprouts, or sprouts. The idea is to mix these foods with fresh vegetables and create different simple dishes based on real food.

Cheeses and vegetable milk are an excellent option to replace traditional dairy products, very easy to make and full of nutrients—coffee with almond milk, chocolate with bitter cocoa, sunflower pâté. The options are endless. The key is variety, complementation, and experimenting in the kitchen.

What about meats?

Like any food of animal origin, Meat has all the essential amino acids -proteins- but these do not come alone. It brings saturated fat, cholesterol, and more digestive work in the combo. In the Hindu tradition of Ayurveda, they speak of being foods with negative *prana*, where the expense for digestion is very high, and they lower the organism's vibration. Observe your body one day you eat meat: how do you feel? How is your digestion? And your mind? What about evacuation? There are no magic formulas: the idea is that you record what is good for you.

In recent times, for various environmental and physiological reasons, it is recommended to reduce meat consumption. The excess of meats, cold cuts, and ultra-processed foods brings metabolic problems, obesity, depression, irritability, diabetes, hypertension, gout, cancer. The FAO - Food and Agriculture Organization of the United Nations contemplates the environmental damage generated by livestock production: deforestation of forests and jungles, loss of oxygen, increasing emissions of greenhouse gases. The greenhouse effect, CO_2, and increased methane gas, and the large water footprint (the waste of water that generates all production) all accelerate the climate change we are already experiencing worldwide.

A separate chapter is the animal abuse of the livestock industry. We are very far from happy cows grazing in the meadow, a typical image of supermarkets or healthy products with green gondolas. The reality has the animals are overcrowded, sick, overdosed on antibiotics, genetically modified to accelerate their growth and increase production. For the world of water: farmed salmon, indiscriminate fishing that is depleting the oceans. They are truths that we find difficult to hear, often uncomfortable. But be it because of the environment, abuse, or body, it is necessary to eat fewer animals.

Become aware that the reality we are living is part of the action. For these reasons, people who choose to consume animal proteins are recommended to lower the consumption frequency to 1 or 2 times a week, improving its quality.

Non-food sources of nutrition

From a more holistic perspective, food is everything that enters through the senses. We nourish ourselves with food for the physical body (which, as we saw, the ideal is to be as real as possible), and there are also the "primary nutrients" - those non-food sources of nutrition that are the ones that satisfy us. They go beyond the plate, nurturing us on a very deep level - feeding the subtlest bodies. Some of those are:

Breathing: breathing is a great tool to calm the mind, fill the body with oxygen and vital energy, detoxify it: eliminating toxins, emotions, stress. Being silent with my eyes closed reconnects me with who I am, with my being, with my gifts and talents. It helps bring the mind to the present moment, focus it.

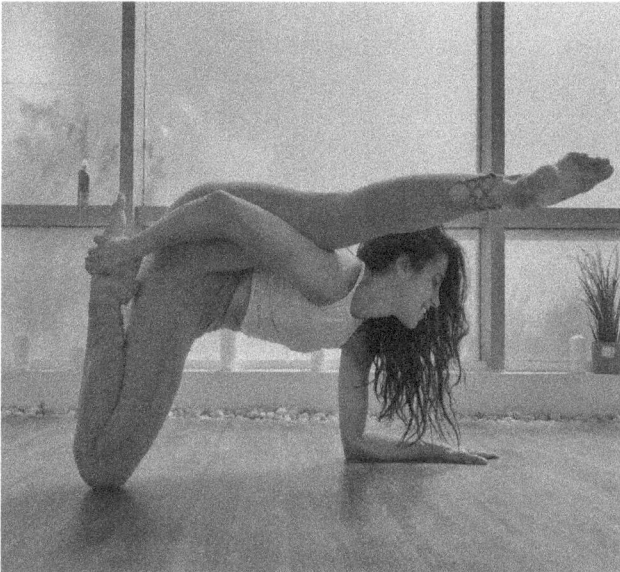

Surrounding yourself with nature: Grounding is a phenomenon of electrical conductivity between the body and the surface of the earth. It is widely studied and applied today by holistic medicine. It generates a feeling of well-being, acting as powerful antioxidants, canceling the inflammation produced by free radicals. It prevents degenerative diseases and premature aging of cells.

Sun: Exposure for 20 min a day helps to synthesize vitamin D and absorb vital energy

Hobbies: What do you like to do?

Physical activity: Build muscle mass, move the body, release endorphins.

Inspirational work: Gifts and talents in service, united to your purpose?

Relationships: Contact with the living, animals, music, song.

The author of "Women Who Run With Wolves" calls them soul food. I use them as fundamental tools in eating plans. They help to return to the center, lower anxiety, generate endorphins, calm the mind, stimulate the creative side, connect with self-care, self-love, and, therefore, with the food we feed our bodies for fuel.

Today, **many people prefer to opt for a plant-based diet** or a vegan diet, rather than diets of animal origin, all to improve **their diet, health, and lifestyle**.

It is always interesting to know more about these healthy lifestyles, but to do this, you must first identify what the **differences are between a plant-based diet and a vegan diet.** This way, you will know which one to choose to make a healthy change to your diet.

Plant-Based is not Veganism

The term "vegan" was created in 1944 by Donald Watson, he was an English defender of animals and, at the same time, founder of The Vegan Society. He created this term to describe people who avoid the use of animals for ethical reasons.

Veganism was expanded to include a diet that excluded the consumption of foods derived from animals, such as eggs, meat, fish, poultry, cheese, and other dairy products. A vegan diet includes vegetables, fruits, grains, nuts, seeds, and legumes.

With time, veganism also became a movement that cared about the environment and health, and not only about ethics and animal welfare.

Thanks to veganism, people have become much more aware of the negative effects of exploiting animals for food and money and the negative effects of consuming a diet rich in animal foods.

History of the "plant-based diet."

During the 1980s, Dr. Colin Campbell introduced the term "plant-based diet" to nutritional science. In this way, it defines a diet low in fat, rich in fiber, and based on plants, which focuses on health and not on consuming animals' ethics.

For a better example, here is a list of products where you will find if you can consume or use them during a vegan and plant-based diet, as well as a whole plant-based meal:

- **Meat, seafood, eggs, and dairy:** you should not consume them during a vegan diet, but on a plant-based diet occasionally

- **Oils:** yes, you can consume them during a vegan and vegetarian diet

- **Whole grains**: if you can consume them during a vegetarian and vegan diet, as well as in a whole plant-based diet.

- **Fruits and vegetables**: if you can consume them in the three types of diets.

- **Legumes:** legumes can also be consumed in all diets.

Differences between a vegetable diet and a vegan diet: what does a plant-based diet mean?

Many people use the term "plant-based" to indicate that they consume a diet that comprises entirely or mainly plant-origin foods. However, some products derived from animals can also be consumed and purchased in smaller quantities.

Other people use the term "raw vegan" to describe their diet as consisting mainly of whole plant foods that are raw or minimally processed (Campbell, 2017).

A person on a diet based on raw whole and plant foods should also avoid consuming processed oils and grains, while these foods can be consumed during a vegan diet.

This is a very important distinction, as there are many processed vegan foods. For example, there are many burgers, types of cheeses, bacon, and even "chicken" nuggets that are vegan but not recommended for a plant-based, whole-food diet.

What does it mean to follow a vegan diet?

Being vegan goes far beyond a simple diet. It also describes the lifestyle that a person chooses to lead daily. Veganism is about living in a way that avoids consuming, using, or exploiting animals as much as realistically possible. The intention is that minimal harm is done to animals through life choices.

Besides avoiding plant-based foods during their diet, people who describe themselves as "vegan" generally avoid buying items made or tested on animals.

These items include clothing, personal care products, shoes, accessories, and household items. For some vegans, this also includes avoiding medications or immunizations that use animal by-products or that have been tested on animals.

Can a person be vegan and vegetarian at the same time?

Many people can start by being vegetarians, avoiding animal products in their diet (mainly for ethical or environmental reasons). These people adapt to a diet based only on plants and whole foods to improve their health and eliminate animal products.

Therefore, you cannot be both simultaneously (since vegetarians only do not eat meat, while vegans do not consume or use any type of animal product), but being vegetarian and being vegan are usually steps within the same process.

Today, a large number of people seek to improve their quality of life through a good diet. For them, the meaning of a "good diet" is based on consuming plant origin products, leaving aside the consumption of food from animals.

On the one hand, there are vegans whose diet is based solely on consuming vegetables. But vegans not only focus on food, but they also avoid buying animal products for ethical reasons.

While on the other hand, there are vegetarians, who are those whose diet is based mainly on the consumption of vegetables, but who at the same time can buy certain products from animals.

With the introduction of food additives, our way of eating has radically changed.

When we read a nutritional label, we come across some terms like these: Tetrazine (E 102), Carmoizine (E 122), and Sodium Benzoate (E 211).

They don't sound like the ingredients our grandmother would use to make food.

They are food additives commonly used in many industrialized foods and beverages.

What are food additives?

Food additives are chemicals that are added to our food for one of the following purposes:

- Add more flavor
- Make the color more attractive
- Nutritionally "enrich" them
- Make them stay on the shelf longer without spoiling.
- Make them sweeter on the palate
- Give a more pleasant texture

But not all food additives that are added to processed food are safe.

The food additives mentioned above were at the center of the debate. Much has been said that they can have effects on children's behavior.

Specifically, there is a study by the *Food Commission* of Great Britain which suggests that food additives labeled with the letter E can cause tantrums and hyperactivity in young children.

Here is a list of the most common food additives.

There are no definitive conclusions about the effects that many food additives and preservatives can cause in the short and long term. But, horror stories can serve as morals to avoid eating food that contains food additives.

A few years ago, in China - July 2013 - it was discovered that chicken feet preserved for 46years with peroxide bleach had been put up for sale.

What, what?

Yes, how you heard it. These chicken feet stayed somewhere for 46 years before being marketed and consumed by children and adults.

Incredible as it may seem, it was.

This extreme case can make us think about what comes out of a package, bag, or package, and we put it in our mouth.

It should also make us think about what the food industry is willing to do to sell its products.

Food additives, colorings, and preservatives are inseparable from almost all processed foods today.

They allow the appearance, smell, and taste to be pleasant to the taste. And yet, what we ingest is a highly artificial flavor.

There is a tremendous amount of money that the food industry invests in processed food.

Behind creating flavors and smells that feel real but are completely artificial, there is a huge effort to make that food sell.

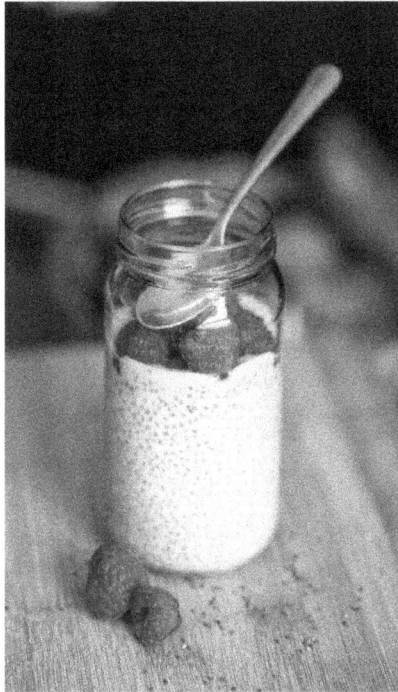

Micha Moss, a reporter for the New York Times, was invited to an unusual experiment.

While gathering information for his book *"Salt, Sugar, and Fat: How the Food Giants Got Us Hooked," he* was invited by Kellogg to their Research and Development Department.

The intention was for him to try some of their flagship products, but free of salt.

This is what the reporter commented:

"I can tell you that it was a terrible experience to taste those things... I couldn't even swallow them.... The most impressive moment was when it was the turn of the cereal without salt. It tasted like metal. "

"Producers use hundreds of substances to disguise the flavors that remain as a result of the production process, " commented Michael Moss.

However, the food industry continues to claim that it is searching for "natural and healthy" formulas, but this is not the product of ethical or reasonable biases of its research and development departments.

Bruce Bradley believes that the food industry has simply identified a new market niche. *"These companies are extremely focused on economic benefits and not on the health of the population."*

"If *the food industry can find a way to sell a product and make a profit on it, I'm sure it will,"* said Bruce Bradley.

So dear friends of this blog, it is unwise to expect the food industry to change and provide us with healthy options.

To do nothing about it would be disastrous for the health of our people.

Instead, you can take close tools to make better decisions regarding your nutrition.

The future has already caught up with us in various ways. Just look at the statistics of overweight in the general population, adolescents, and children in Latin America and the United States.

The numbers for diabetes, cancer, and heart disease are also outrageous. We have to do something about it, each one of us.

It is not too late to change, nor do you have to wait for change to come by itself.

The best advice I can give you is to:

The next time you find yourself in front of a package of industrialized food, ask yourself if it is the best option for you and your family.

Is it the food that will contribute to my well-being, or will it just make me feel good for a short time, needing more and more?

The answer is obvious, and with that in mind, you have to make smarter decisions.

You can learn to read labels and choose fresher options, free of hormones and dyes, and do not contain food additives dangerous to health.

You can also cook more. That by itself will reduce your risk of getting sick from something serious and help you maintain a healthier weight.

Let's not let that irresistible pre-made craving win us over. We can make the change ourselves. We should not wait for the authorities to take care of our health. It is up to you and me to do it.

Chapter 3: What Makes Plant-Based Model Most Exciting?

Eating a diet where the bases are vegetables, fruits, cereals, legumes, and seeds can provide many benefits for your health, economy, and lifestyle. It also has positive repercussions on the environment and food safety, being one of the most sustainable.

But what are these benefits?

Helps maintain a healthy weight

In a study conducted by the International Journal of Obesity and Metabolic Disorders, it was found that people who follow a plant-based diet, which includes a variety of vegetables, whole fruits, whole grains, legumes or legumes, nuts, and seeds, have more likely to have a healthy fat percentage and less likely to be overweight, staying within the Body Mass Index ranges for average weight. On the contrary, consuming saturated fat from foods of animal origin, excess protein from meats, and a low fiber diet are related to a high body mass index and more significant body fat accumulation.

Switching to a plant-based diet is suitable for both the soul and the body. By making the switch, we renounce our selfish consumption of scarce resources to feed the world. We condemn the cruel and inhumane practice of raising animals in abominable conditions to feed our taste for meat. A plant-based diet causes the least amount of harm and suffering to other living things, which is undoubtedly good for the soul.

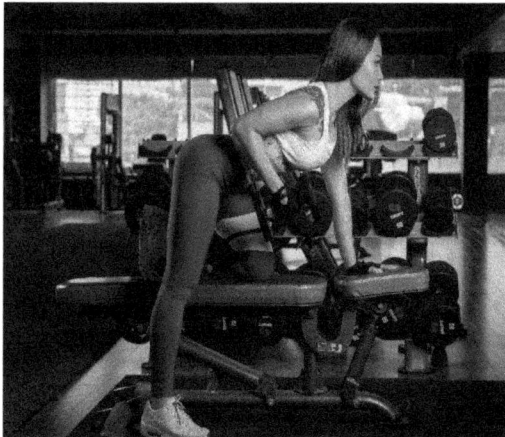

Nothing could be simpler than fresh fruits and vegetables from the bounty of the earth. And as we become more aware of the negative impacts a meat-based diet has on the environment, personal health, and world hunger, plant-based alternatives are becoming more visible and widely available in the world. Even some fast-food restaurants now offer vegan and vegetarian menus.

Prevents against chronic degenerative diseases

Several epidemiological studies have shown that adults who eat a plant-based diet have a lower incidence of many chronic diseases controlled by diet and eating habits, such as high blood pressure, type 2 diabetes mellitus, and cardiovascular diseases. People who follow this type of diet are more likely to improve insulin sensitivity, reduce cholesterol and triglyceride levels in the blood, and decrease the dose of medications taken, as appropriate.

Promotes safe food consumption

Animal foods such as meat, dairy, and farm-raised fish can contain hormones, steroids, and other toxic residues from their eating and processing. Consuming organic products and reducing consumption of animal foods can help limit exposure to these toxins.

A plant-based diet has been shown to reduce the risk of many chronic diseases, such as obesity, coronary artery disease, high blood pressure, diabetes, colon, breast, prostate, stomach, lung cancer, and esophagus. A plant-based diet can also relieve menopausal symptoms and provide relief from various digestive ailments.

According to the US Centers for Disease Control (CDC), 76 million people are affected by foodborne illness each year. Although any food can become contaminated, the most frequent and severe foodborne illness cases come from meat and other animal products.

Saves money on the purchase of food products

According to a study comparing the cost of various types of healthy eating, those who follow a plant-based diet can save about $750 per year. Consuming seasonal fruits and vegetables, whole grains, legumes such as beans, lentils, chickpeas, soybeans, and oilseeds such as peanuts, sunflower seeds, and squash is economical and also highly nutritious. Purchasing our food in local markets and central supply centers, and using food properly to avoid a large amount of food waste or waste, are also important ways to reduce costs.

It is friendly with the environment

The great demand for animal origin products is one of the leading causes of jungles and forests' deforestation. These spaces are used to raise animals and grow the food they require, being almost 30% of the land area is used to raise livestock. Farm animals also contribute to greenhouse gases, which are linked to global warming.

The United Nations FAO report in 2006 unequivocally stated that the industrial farming of animals for meat production has a more significant impact on global warming than all the planes, trains, buses, and cars on the planet combined.

Raising animals for meat consumes large amounts of water. According to the article "How Our Food Choices Can Help Save the Environment" by Steve Boyan, Ph.D. (www.earthsave.org), eliminating just one pound of beef from your diet can save the most water that could be saved when showering entirely for six months!

Runoff from factory farms containing chemicals and animal waste, one of the biggest threats to water quality today, has polluted more than 173,000 miles of rivers and streams in the U.S. (Environmental Protection Agency)

Meat production is a costly and inefficient use of food resources. According to John Robbins in Diet for a New America, the grain required to feed cattle in the United States for one day is enough to provide every person on earth with two loaves of bread. The fact is that more people can be fed a plant-based diet than a diet containing meat and dairy.

Economizes the use of energy resources

Plant-based foods require less energy, space, and water to produce, prepare, and store than animal-based foods. Animal protein uses 100 times more water than the same amount of protein from grains. Besides, many plant-based foods do not require refrigeration and can be eaten raw, reducing energy use for preparation and storage.

Eating a complete and varied plant-based diet can help prevent nutritional deficiencies

The deficiencies of **macronutrients** (proteins, carbohydrates, and fats) and **micronutrients** (vitamins and minerals), which are compounds necessary to maintain a good state of health, cause a complex series of symptoms and signs, characteristic for each nutrient, and that evolves in 3 stages: depletion of reserves, biochemical dysfunction in the body and, finally, a deficiency or deficiency state.

What is called a "nutritional deficiency"?

A deficiency occurs when the body does not receive enough nutrients for all the physiological processes that support health and life to be carried out correctly. When there is a deficiency, the organs and tissues develop problems that, over time, can be serious.

The list of nutrients that we must incorporate, each in a specific dose, is long so that deficiencies can affect a large part of the population.

Deficiency symptoms are highly variable, depending on the nutrient in question, but can be detected in a physical examination and physiological symptoms through studies and blood tests.

What are macro and micronutrients?

Among the macronutrients, we find those that provide energy (calories) and "building materials" for body tissues: carbohydrates, fats, and proteins. They are needed in large quantities (grams).

Micronutrients are involved in physiological processes but are required in smaller amounts (milligrams). They are minerals and vitamins.

What factors can favor the appearance of nutritional deficiencies?

Monotonous diet: Not eating in a varied and healthy way, or always eating the same foods, represents a risk of suffering from a deficiency since there are no foods that can provide all the nutrients 100%.

Restrictive diets: Following diet plans to lose weight in which many foods are prohibited and are very low in calories, or that are based on the consumption of a single food (for example, "the apple diet") can cause significant nutritional deficiencies, which put health at risk.

Excessive consumption of industrialized food and fast food: Packaged or industrialized products, especially those based on refined flours and sugars, barely contain micronutrients concerning the amount of energy (calories) they provide. The same thing happens with fast food: you consume a lot of calories but few nutrients.

Special nutritional needs: During adolescence, pregnancy, and lactation, the body has increased needs for many nutrients. Athletes and people under physical and mental stress also have specific or increased needs for certain nutrients. Consult with a specialist to know your requirements according to your situation.

Specific diseases: People with an intestinal disorder, for example, may have difficulty absorbing certain nutrients, so they must obtain them in greater quantities from food. Many medications can also affect the absorption of nutrients.

Consumption of stimulants: High consumption of alcohol, coffee, refined and sugary foods, nicotine, and other harmful stimulants harm the absorption of nutrients and lead to a deficiency.

Stress: It can cause loss of appetite and gastrointestinal disorders, and these factors, in turn, promote deficiency.

How can a plant-based diet help prevent and treat nutritional deficiencies?

It is essential to know that most of the nutrients and substances vital to maintaining health can be found in vegetables or enriched foods. Still, it is imperative that if you eat a plant-based diet, it is appropriate for each person's needs, complete and varied.

Protein deficiency

Getting the minimum protein is not a problem for most people on a plant-based diet. There is a problem of excess: 80% of people eat more than they need due to meat's excessive consumption.

For adults, the protein requirements per kilogram of weight are the same for both genders. The accepted value for a safe intake level is 0.75 g per kg per day, in terms of easily digestible proteins (mung beans, chickpeas, tempeh, peanut butter, almonds, and other nuts, spirulina).

Symptoms of a lack of protein can be the following:

• Exhaustion and feeling of lack of energy.

• Loss of muscle volume.

• Increased tendency to suffer infections.

• Fluid retention (seen, for example, in abdominal swelling and heavy legs).

The food solution consists of consuming a large portion of legumes daily (beans, lentils, chickpeas, broad beans, beans, soybeans, and their derivatives) and supplements of cereals, nuts, and seeds.

Carbohydrate and fat deficiency

It is sporadic for these macronutrients to be deficient, except in cases of severe malnutrition.

To prevent deficiencies in these nutrients, a plant-based diet should be varied, including vegetables, fruits, whole grains, and vegetable fats, such as seeds, nuts, and avocado, inadequate amounts depending on each person's needs.

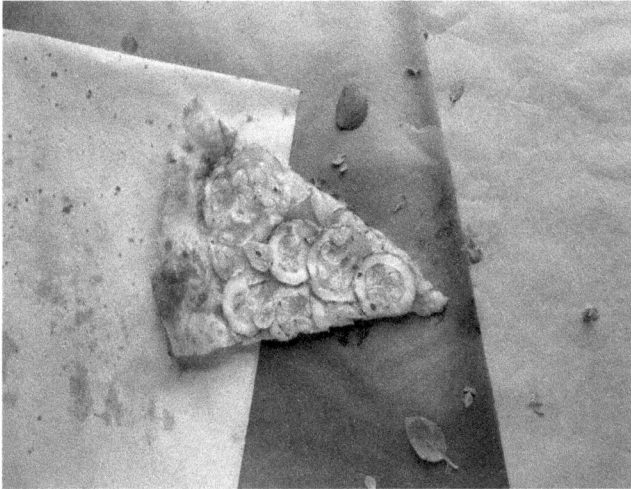

Lack of iron

Iron is a mineral needed, among other things, that the red blood cells to carry oxygen. This mineral deficiency is widespread, especially among women of childbearing age and people with gastrointestinal disorders.

Typical symptoms of deficiency are:

• Drowsiness

• Concentration problems

• Paleness, dizziness, and headaches

• Brittle nails and hair loss

The dietary solution to iron deficiency is to increase foods that contain iron in abundance, such as lentils and other legumes, sesame or sesame, green leafy vegetables, whole grains, nuts.

To better assimilate this iron provided by plant foods, it is important to combine it with foods rich in vitamin C (fresh fruits and vegetables) and avoid consuming foods containing caffeine with those rich in iron.

Vitamin B12 deficiency

Those who follow a strict plant-based diet and do not supplement vitamin B12 may suffer from a deficiency. This nutrient is essential for the production of red blood cells and, therefore, for oxygen transport. The functioning of the nervous system and energy metabolism also depend on B12.

Older people can also be deficient due to poor intestinal absorption. The following symptoms recognize the deficiency:

• Tiredness, dejection.

• Concentration problems.

• Paleness and anemia.

• Alteration of the mucous membranes.

• Numbness and tingling in the extremities.

• Feeling of disorientation.

There are three options for vitamin B12 supplementation: take a daily supplement of 25-100 mcg or a weekly supplement of 2,000 mcg, or consume enough foods enriched with this vitamin.

Calcium deficiency

Calcium not only has a crucial role in our bones but is also present in the blood, as it plays a vital role in coagulation. It also works as an electrolyte: both in the brain, where it participates in sending and receiving nerve signals between neurons, and in muscles, which is essential for their contraction and relaxation. Also, it is necessary for correct cardiac function and the secretion of some hormones.

Calcium deficiency symptoms:

• Increases the risk of osteoporosis due to loss of bone mass.

• Appearance of muscle spasms, cramps, numbness.

• In severe cases, palpitations, and disorientation.

In a plant-based diet, calcium is found in the entire cruciferous family (broccoli, cauliflower, cabbage, kale, watercress, radishes), in nuts such as almonds, seeds such as sesame, legumes (especially soybeans) and beans), tofu (especially curdled with calcium salts) and other derivatives of soy, and enriched vegetable drinks (commonly called vegetable milk).

What to do when you have a nutritional deficiency?

- To prevent or treat any deficiencies, you should consider the following:
- Improve your diet. You must eat in a balanced way with a good variety of foods. For that, you must include legumes, fruits, vegetables, whole grain products, and healthy fats in your eating plan.
- Make sure that you consume several servings a day of vegetable foods, according to your characteristics and needs. Consult a health professional who can guide you.
- Avoid fast food, snacks, and "ready to eat" products. It is advisable to include at least three servings of raw or fresh food daily.
- —If you are pregnant or a nursing mother, talk to your doctor to cover possible deficiencies or an increased need for certain nutrients.
- Avoid alcohol, caffeine, and nicotine.
- Control stress.

Many natural disasters cannot be prevented; others are the consequence of human actions.

As the name implies, natural disasters are those sudden and violent events caused by the natural processes of the planet, that is, by the interaction mainly of abiotic elements. Most of them cannot be controlled and have nothing to do with human activity. However, in recent decades, natural disasters have increased in frequency and severity, linked to human activities that degrade the environment, such as gas emissions. Greenhouse effects, deforestation, and pollution that generate, among others, phenomena such as climate change, desertification, loss of biodiversity, and other accelerated phenomena that, although they have always occurred and are part of the earth's natural processes, have only increased their impacts and therefore the risks they pose for people, countries, and companies.

The World Economic Forum has reported that among the top 10 risks for businesses and countries are natural disasters, disasters caused by human action, climate change, loss of biodiversity, heat waves, and bushfires. All of these have, to a certain extent, a close relationship with food. Since jungle and forest areas are being exchanged for induced grasslands or farmlands, natural water reserves are being emptied to meet the demand for this activity that requires 27 % of the planet's water and, mainly, it is an activity that generates a third of the anthropogenic emissions of greenhouse gases on the planet.

Faced with the climate emergency that is coming, or that some of us consider that we already have, it is necessary to do everything possible to reduce the increase in temperature through the reduction of greenhouse gas emissions, so it is crucial that policies focused on climate action, establish food policies to minimize emissions from this sector, with livestock, poultry, and fish farming being the ones that emit the most greenhouse gases together in the food sector, and the change in diets has a potential greater in the reduction of emissions than the technological changes that may occur in this sector; however, most countries have ignored this strategy in their action plans.

Therefore, to reduce the risk posed by natural disasters, a change in the food paradigms towards more sustainable diets must be part of national and corporate strategies to prevent and even mitigate action.

Thanks to social networks, information like the one we present in this blog reaches more people. However, it is also necessary to put it into practice. Since industrial canteens or restaurants near work centers feed a large proportion of the economically active population, it is their responsibility not only to show information on the environmental impacts of their gastronomic offer but to promote sustainable diets as a rule and not the exception of its dishes.

How can I make my diet more nutritious and complete?

We have always heard that to have a healthy diet, it is essential to eat fruits and vegetables, so much so that the dietary guidelines of all countries, important health institutions, and even the governments of different nations have promoted the abundant consumption of vegetables typical of their region— in all stages of life.

Regarding the recommendation of how many vegetables to eat, we found that the idea is to include 3 to 5 different vegetables per day, or two cups of mixed vegetables, and 3 to 4 pieces of fruit, or 1 ½ cups of mixed fruits, for the day, trying to make them of different colors and textures, to add not only more nutritional properties but also different textures and flavors to the dishes. But how does including a good variety of vegetables help make my diet more nutritious?

The more vegetables you add to your dishes, the more color they will have, and this is important because...

Each "color" provides different nutrients:

Red

Red vegetables and fruits owe their color to lycopene. Lycopene is a natural vegetable pigment, belonging to the group of carotenoids, which provides red color to tomatoes, bell peppers, and fruits such as watermelon, strawberries, red or pink grapefruit. This carotenoid has antioxidant, anti-cancer, and anti-cell aging properties.

Green

All green vegetables provide greater or lesser amounts of lutein and β-carotene (belonging to the group of carotenoids). Vegetables rich in lutein include spinach, lettuce, and Brussels sprouts. Also, these three are high in β-carotene along with broccoli and peas.

Yellow

The natural plant pigments responsible for the yellow color of fruits and vegetables belong to flavonoids. These have been linked to antioxidant and anti-cancer properties and the prevention of cardiovascular and cerebrovascular diseases. On the other hand, zeaxanthin is a carotenoid (responsible for the yellow color) found in high concentrations in corn.

Orange

Orange vegetables owe their color to α-carotene and β-carotene, which belong to the group of carotenoids. Among vegetables, the best sources of α-carotene and β-carotene are carrots and pumpkin. While melon, mango, and orange are the fruits with the highest contribution of these carotenoids. It is followed by other fruits and vegetables such as potatoes, citrus fruits (grapefruit and tangerine), peaches, papaya, and apricots. Carotenoids are precursors of vitamin A (provitamin A), have the antioxidant capacity, provide benefits for vision and skin, promote the immune system, and prevent cardiovascular diseases.

Vegetables provide a lot of nutrients but few calories

Vegetables and fruits are foods whose major nutritional contributions are carbohydrates, fiber, water, vitamins, and minerals. One of the greatest benefits of consuming vegetables and fruits is that they contain very few calories, but their nutritional contribution is abundant. For example:

- 1 cup of broccoli = 31 kcal
- 1 cup of raw carrot = 50 kcal
- 1 cup of lettuce = 14 kcal
- 1 cup of chopped melon = 53 kcal
- 1 cup of strawberries = 49 kcal

We can get a different variety of vegetables and fruits per season

January - Chard, garlic, eggplant, beets, zucchini, onion, cabbage, cauliflower, peas, green chili, green beans, corn, spinach, tomato, lettuce, potato, cucumber, tomato, carrot, strawberry, guava, hibiscus, lime, lemon, mandarin, melon, orange, pineapple, papaya, banana, grapefruit, tejocote, Chinese pomegranate, and tamarind.

February - Chard, garlic, aubergine, beet, zucchini, onion, cabbage, cauliflower, chayote, pea, green chili, green bean, spinach, tomato, lettuce, potato, cucumber, radish, tomato, carrot, strawberry, Chinese pomegranate, mamey, lemon, tangerine, papaya, watermelon, tamarind, grapefruit, pineapple, and mango.

March - Chard, garlic, zucchini, onion, cabbage, cauliflower, chayote, pea, green chili, green bean, corn, spinach, tomato, nopal, potato, cucumber, radish, carrot, mamey, lemon, strawberry, tangerine, orange, papaya, banana, watermelon, grapefruit, tamarind, and mango.

April - Chard, garlic, beet, zucchini, onion, cabbage, cauliflower, chayote, pea, green chili, green bean, spinach, tomato, lettuce, nopal, potato, cucumber, radish, tomato, carrot, orange, papaya, pineapple, watermelon, banana, grapefruit, tamarind, strawberry, lemon, mango, mamey, and melon.

May - Chard, garlic, eggplant, beet, zucchini, onion, cabbage, cauliflower, pea, green chili, green bean, corn, spinach, tomato, lettuce, potato, cucumber, tomato, carrot, plum, strawberry, apricot, lemon, mamey mango, melon, pear, orange, papaya, watermelon, grapefruit, banana, and pineapple.

June - Chard, avocado, garlic, watercress, zucchini, onion, cabbage, cauliflower, chayote, pea, green bean, corn, spinach, tomato, lettuce, nopal, potato, cucumber, tomato, purslane, carrot, lemon, plum, apricot, peach, fig, mango, mamey, apple, melon, pear, pineapple, banana, grape, watermelon, and grapefruit.

July - Chard, avocado, garlic, zucchini, onion, cabbage, cauliflower, pea, green chili, green bean, corn, tomato, lettuce, nopal, potato, cucumber, tomato, carrot, pear, plum, peach, red pomegranate, lemon, fig, apple, mango, melon, quince, papaya, pineapple, banana, watermelon, prickly pear, grapefruit, and grapes.

August - Avocado, beet, zucchini, onion, cabbage, cauliflower, pea, poblano pepper, green pepper, green bean, corn, tomato, lettuce, nopal, potato, cucumber, tomato, carrot, plum, peach, capulin, red pomegranate, fig, guava, mango, lemon, apple, quince, pear, papaya, pineapple, banana, grapefruit, tuna, and grapes.

September - Chard, avocado, beet, onion, cabbage, cauliflower, pea, poblano pepper, green pepper, green bean, corn, spinach, tomato, lettuce, potato, cucumber, tomato, carrot, red pomegranate, quince, orange, papaya, pear, perón, banana, watermelon, grapefruit, tuna, peach, guava, lemon, apple, and melon.

October - Chard, avocado, aubergine, beet, zucchini, pumpkin, onion, cabbage, cauliflower, pea, chili, poblano, green chili, green bean, corn, spinach, tomato, lettuce, potato, cucumber, tomato, carrot, tangerine, apple, quince, orange, papaya, pear, perón, banana, tejocote, grape, grapefruit, lemon, guava, red pomegranate, peach, and sapodilla.

November - Chard, avocado, aubergine, beet, zucchini, pumpkin, onion, cabbage, cauliflower, pea, chili, poblano, green chili, green bean, corn, spinach, tomato, lettuce, potato, cucumber, tomato, carrot, grapes, grapefruit, hawthorn, banana, pear, papaya, orange, tangerine, lime, lemon, guava, jicama, Chinese pomegranate, and strawberry.

December - Chard, avocado, beet, pumpkin, cabbage, cauliflower, spinach, tomato, lettuce, potato, cucumber, tomato, carrot, cane, strawberry, custard apple, sapodilla, Chinese pomegranate, jicama, guava, lime, lemon, orange, mandarin, papaya, pear, banana, hawthorn, pineapple, black sapote, and grapefruit.

They can be prepared in different ways and give different textures to the dishes.

Stews: You can fry different vegetables with a little vegetable oil and add spices, herbs, or sauces.

Soups, creams, and purees: They allow you to mix different vegetables with broths and spices.

Sauces: You can prepare fresh or spicy sauces, such as guacamole, red sauce, toreada sauce, etc.

Green smoothies: Combining various types of vegetables and fruits in a blender is an easy way to reap their benefits.

Salads: There is a wide variety of salads, and you can add as many vegetables as you like. Accompany them with seeds and vinaigrettes to give them more flavor and texture.

How to lose weight with a plant-based diet?

Do you know how to lose weight with a *plant-based* diet? Do you know what a plant-based diet consists of?

Can you imagine eating pasta, rice, chickpeas, legumes, and potatoes and losing weight? Do you believe me if I tell you that you can lose all your excess weight by eating this type of food?

This is exactly what I have been doing for almost a year now, and I have lost over 40 lbs without starving or craving for food.

I have also experienced dramatic positive changes in my energy level, mood, and addiction to certain foods.

Do you want to know where "the trick" is?

Let me tell you.

For years I have been convinced that to lose weight, I had to stop eating carbohydrates: bread, pasta, rice, legumes, etc.

In fact, throughout my life, I have followed many diets based on this principle. Every time I had to lose weight, my diet was based on eating salads, boiled vegetables, lean meat, chicken, turkey, eggs, and grilled fish.

It is true that, when I managed to maintain this type of diet beyond a few weeks, I lost some weight, but always with great suffering.

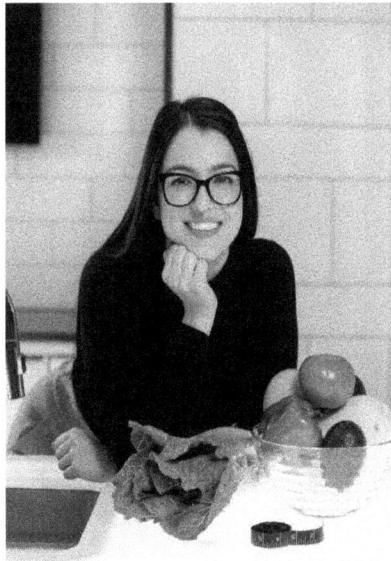

This suffering materialized in the form of being hungry, anxious about food, having a hard time in social situations, and constantly being in a bad mood.

She did lose some weight (only at first, then quickly regained it), but she could only enjoy it when she bought new clothes in a smaller size. The rest of the time – the process until she lost several kilos in weight – was a real torture, a constant struggle between what she wanted to eat and what she should eat.

But as I had always been told that "to be thin you have to suffer, unless you have privileged genetics," here I was, constantly suffering, putting all the willpower I had on my part to control what I ate regularly.

Have you had an experience similar to mine?

After more than 20 years of low carbohydrate diets without permanent results, I radically changed my diet and surprise about one year ago! I started to lose weight without anxiety, without having a hard time, and without suffering. In addition, I was feeling better and better, with an amount of energy that I had not had in years.

But today, I am not going to tell you about all the changes that I have personally experienced. Today what I want to tell you is what this wonderful diet has radically changed my life.

What does it mean to follow a *plant-based* diet?

A *plant-based* diet consists of consuming foods of plant origin.

1. Base your diet on the consumption of plant-based foods

2. Eliminate as much as possible (or better, completely) foods of animal origin

3. Eliminate processed foods

4. Eliminate as much as possible (or better, completely) refined foods

1. Base your diet on the consumption of plant-based foods

Vegetables, vegetables, fruits, cereals, whole grains, legumes, aromatic herbs, nuts, and seeds are the foundations of a plant-based diet.

These are the recommended food groups to consume daily when following a *plant-based* diet.

The combinations are endless, and the belief that eating this type of food makes you fat is a total fallacy.

That which we have been told all our lives that chickpeas, potatoes, or pasta are fattening is false. What makes us fat is the meat and the chorizo with which we cook the chickpeas, the oil we use to fry the potatoes and the cheese and the fried tomato that we use to make a pasta dish.

So, the first step to eating a *plant-based* diet is to start dispelling myths and basing our diet on *plant-based* foods.

2. Eliminate as much as possible (or better completely) foods of animal origin

Animal foods are packed with saturated fat, cholesterol, and sodium. Even those foods that traditionally have told us that they have less fat (such as chicken or fish) still have much more fat than most plant origin foods.

Take a look at these examples per 100 grams of food:

- Chicken thigh: 11.2 g total fat (3.67 g saturated fat)

- Chicken breast: 6.2 g total fat (1.91 g saturated fat)

- Salmon: 12.1 g of total fat (2.10 g of saturated fat)

- Canned lentils: 0.7 g total fat (0.1 g saturated fat)

- Potatoes: 0.11 g of total fat (0.03 g of saturated fat)

- Brown rice: 2.20 g of total fat (0.61 g of saturated fat)

Also, many foods of animal origin, such as red meat and processed meat, are hyper-concentrated foods related to food addiction, directly contribute to overweight and obesity, and the main global nutritional guidelines recommend reducing or eliminating their consumption to the negative implications they have for health.

There are other reasons why you should stop consuming animal foods that go beyond weight loss and health.

3. Eliminate as much as possible (or better completely) processed foods

Processed foods are those foods that have changed due to some degree of industrial processing.

While some foods have undergone minimal processing, such as cooked legumes or bagged lettuce, other products have been ultra-processed, such as pre-cooked dishes or industrial pastries.

Processed foods have been manipulated to improve their preservation, taste, and appearance to a greater or lesser extent. High amounts of fat, salt, sugars, colorants, preservatives, and sweeteners are added to do this.

These added substances facilitate overweight, create addiction, and substantially reduce the nutritional quality of food. This is the reason why it is not advisable to consume this type of food.

Suppose you want to follow a healthy diet and take advantage of all the benefits of plant foods. In that case, it is important to eliminate processed foods as much as possible, especially those with added ingredients such as oils, salt, sugars, sweeteners, preservatives, and colorings. The more ingredients a product has, the more negative for your health.

4. Eliminate the most (or better completely) refined foods

Refined foods have been subjected to different types of manipulation until reaching their final form, destroying, during the process, part of the nutritional value of the original foods.

For example, white flour, sugar, oils, and hydrogenated fats have undergone a refinement process in which fiber and other beneficial natural nutrients have been removed. This refinement converts "white" foods into hyper-concentrated foods that negatively affect our health and promote food addiction.

In turn, the absence of fiber from refined foods is bad news. Fiber is essential for our health and helps us, among other things, to keep the intestines healthy, prevent colon cancer, improve satiety, and control weight.

One goal of eating a plant-based diet is to cut down on refined foods, starting with the most harmful like white flour, sugar, and highly refined oils like palm oil and hydrogenated fats.

5. How can you start losing weight without hunger or anxiety?

This phrase has guided me for years: **"If a strategy doesn't work for you, change it."**

If you are overweight and you have tried various weight-loss strategies, and they have not worked for you, the only thing I can tell you is: **change your strategy -> switch to a plant-based diet**.

To do this, follow these points:

1. Base your diet on plant origin foods: fruits, vegetables, legumes, cereals, nuts, and seeds.

2. Eliminate or minimize animal origin foods: red meat, poultry, dairy, eggs, and fish.

3. Ditch the processed foods and choose those foods that come directly from nature.

4. Eliminate or minimize refined foods and choose unrefined ones like whole grains and whole grains.

Following a *plant-based* diet will allow you to lose weight without starving or anxiety. How?

- **You will lose weight** because you will reduce the caloric density of the food you eat,

- **you will not starve** because you will give your body the volume and adequate nutrients it needs and,

- **You will not have anxiety** because you will eliminate all those foods directly related to anxiety and food addiction.

Plant-Based Diet – Let's recap some science

The year is nearing its end, so it is time to re-visit **the most important learning moments** and prepare for a **2021 full of progress and positive changes** for our health, that of the living beings that surround us, and our planet.

In that spirit, I **compiled three studies that came to light this year**, indicating, on a scientific basis, that the plant-based diet is essential for not only the prevention of diseases but also their reversal.

Up to 1/3 Of Premature Deaths Can Be Prevented

According to Harvard scientists, **at least a third of premature deaths can be prevented by adopting a vegetarian diet**. Dr. Walter Willett of Harvard Medical School said that a plant-based diet's benefits had been widely underestimated.

He suggested that recent figures from the Office for National Statistics estimate that **around 200,000 lives could have been saved** annually if people had cut meat from their diet.

On the other hand, Professor David Jenkins of the University of Toronto also mentioned that **humans would benefit from eating a diet similar to apes.**

Dr. Neal Barnard, Chairman of the Committee for Responsible Medicine, mentioned that people **need to wake up to vegetarian and vegan diets' powerful benefits.**

"The low-fat vegan diet is better than any other diet I've ever seen in improving diabetes," *Barnard said.*

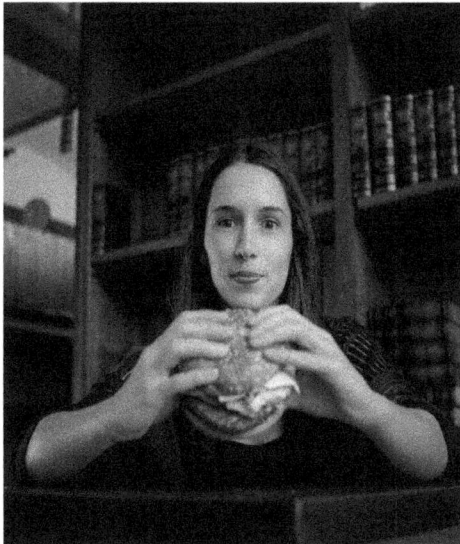

Plant-Derived Fats Healthier Than Animal Fats

The published study by the **Harvard TH Chan School of Public Health suggests that fats from plants are healthier than their counterparts from animals**, at the least in terms of monosaturated fats are concerned.

The monounsaturated fats in plants, found in foods like avocados, nuts, and seeds, are associated with a lower risk of death from cardiovascular disease. On the other hand, monounsaturated fats present in animal products such as meat and derivatives are associated with a greater risk.

People who consumed high amounts of plant **fats had** a **16% lower risk of dying,** while subjects who consumed large amounts of **animal fats showed a 21% higher risk** than those who did not consume these fat sources.

"We have observed a beneficial role of monounsaturated fats in the prevention of cardiovascular diseases when the source of these fats are plants," said Marta Guasch-Ferre, a research associate at The Harvard TH Chan School of Public Health.

Adhering to A Plant-Based Diet Reduces Risk of Obesity

According to a **study** conducted by the European Association for the Study of Obesity, **predominantly adhering to a plant-based diet reduces the risk of obesity in mature and elderly adults.**

During the study, the researchers created a 'plant-based index,' rewarding those who consumed large amounts of plants, such as vegetables, fruits, nuts, and subtracting points from those who consumed animal origin products.

At the end of the study, participants who **consumed higher amounts of plant foods** were **shown to have lower levels of body fat mass,**

*"Our study shows that a diet focused primarily on plants is beneficial in preventing overweight and obesity in mature adults,"*Zhangling Chen, part of the investigation team, said.

The Plant-Based Model

This model establishes food and nutritional guidance criteria that help guarantee a healthy dining room.

The food offered by the business, industrial, community canteens, etc., must be designed to improve employees' food and nutrition since they are the most valuable asset of any company, resulting in wellness programs in the workplace very important for talent retention.

Benefiting employees and providing them with a healthy diet reduces absenteeism and notably improves their work capacity and commitment, and the company finding a way to retain and motivate staff.

In what way the plant-based diet model helps us? Promotion and education for health in food matters, to meet the need for nutritional well-being and healthy eating in the workplace?

1. The consumption of many vegetables and fruits, preferably raw, regional, and seasonal, should be promoted:

I want to touch on the importance of consuming a wide variety of plant foods for health, a source of carotenes, vitamins, mostly A and C, folic acid, minerals, and dietary fiber, and give color and texture to the dishes. Besides, as they are low-calorie density foods, they can be added to the preparations in greater quantities, receiving all their nutritional benefits without significantly increasing the dish's total calories.

2. The consumption of cereals, preferably whole grains or their derivatives, and tubers should be recommended:

Whole grains and tubers stand out for their contribution of dietary fiber and energy, important for satisfactorily and productively fulfilling daily work shifts, especially in those heavy activities or those with high physical impacts, such as construction and agriculture.

3. The recovery of the consumption of the wide variety of beans and diversification with other legumes should be promoted: lentils, beans, chickpeas, and peas, due to their fiber and protein content:

The legumes are vital for global food health, being very cheap and sustainable production for the environment. In addition, its nutritional qualities stand out that they contain around double the amount of protein found in whole grain cereals, and when combined with foods rich in vitamin C, such as citrus fruits and green vegetables, the high iron content of the Legumes can make them a powerful food to replenish iron stores.

Legumes are also a versatile food that can be prepared in many ways and are an excellent alternative to the consumption of protein of animal origin, especially for collaborators with alternative ways of feeding, dietary restrictions, or who suffer from chronic degenerative diseases, since Being of plant origin, legumes do not contain saturated fat or cholesterol, but are rich in protein and fiber.

4. Moderation should be recommended in the consumption of foods of animal origin due to their high content of cholesterol and saturated fats:

In Mexico, the main causes of mortality from illnesses continue to be related to an unhealthy diet and lifestyle: obesity and overweight, diabetes mellitus, and heart disease. The model emphasizes reducing the consumption of animal origin foods since, in most cases, they are the focal point of the dishes served in dining rooms. Still, they represent a risk due to their high content of saturated fat and cholesterol.

5. The importance of varying the diet and exchanging the foods within each group should be emphasized:

One of the important characteristics of a correct diet is variety. The inclusion of different foods in each dish or preparation, mostly vegetable, fresh, seasonal, and regional foods, gives diversity to the diet in terms of flavors and textures and increases its nutritional value and its health benefits.

6. Hygienic practices in food preparation should be emphasized:

Especially in the current situation, it is extremely important to emphasize and implement correct hygiene measures in food preparation stations and all areas of business canteens, such as washing and disinfecting vegetables and fruits, boiling or chlorinating water, washing and properly cook food of animal origin, or that due to its handling characteristics is possible and necessary to ensure its safety, as well as hygiene in the kitchen environment, personal hygiene, cleaning of utensils and food storage.

7. The ideal way to optimize the cost-benefit derived from the selection, preparation, and preservation of food should be indicated:

There is preparation, cooking, storage, and more sustainable disposal techniques, thus improving the dishes' quality, saving food and energy resources, and reducing waste.

8. Local and regional foods should be identified and reassessed, and the use of local culinary techniques that do not harm health should be recommended. The consumption of foods prepared with natural condiments and spices from the traditional cuisine of each region will be promoted:

One of the current trends that food services are taking up is preparing food with regional and traditional techniques and inputs, typical of each state. These food preparation methods promote locally produced food, rescue traditional dishes, and implement healthier cooking methods, improving their nutritional quality and, consequently, the health of those who consume them. Also, they are dishes that are much more sustainable.

These are just some of the important points illustrated, which will considerably improve employees' quality of life inside and outside of work, increasing their enthusiasm and productivity if implemented in business, industrial, community canteens, etc. Do you already carry them out in your company?

Athletes who #MadeTheShift

More and more athletes improve their physical performance by reducing their consumption of foods of animal origin.

The list is very large:

- Carl Lewis - 100m Runner 9 Olympic Gold Medals
- Venus Williams - Tennis Player
- Novak Djokovic - Tennis Player
- Lewis Hamilton - F1 Driver

- Colin Kaepernick - NFL

- Tom Brady - NFL

- Lionel Messi - Footballer

- Sergio Aguero - Footballer

- Kyrie Irving - NBA

- Scot Jurek - 20 ultramarathons

- and many more

Game Changers

Recently, James Cameron's new film: The Game Changers, was shown at film festivals, in which he presents the story of athletes who benefit from a 100% plant-based diet to compete at their best.

The player **Carlos Cuéllar, a vegan since 2014**, tells VICE about this: "I have found that I recover my efforts better, I have more elasticity, and I have more strength for longer." Also, he adds: "I have to do double the exercises in the gym to feel tired."

The main reason for taking this type of diet in athletes is to improve performance. They feel lighter and more energetic. Your results improve and your health also overall. Vegetable proteins are higher in fiber and have a lower content of saturated fat.

To supplement legumes with nuts and cereals throughout the day in order to increase absorption and facilitate the digestion of vegetable protein.

An athlete who follows a **plant-based diet** must "take care of blood creatine levels and ensure adequate levels of vitamin B12, calcium, omega three, and iron." For this reason, he recommends "going to a nutritionist who takes into account your lifestyle and calculates the appropriate amounts of macro and micro-nutrients."

In summary, some of the benefits of a plant-based diet:

- Higher performance

- Lower blood pressure

- Less likely to test positive for prohibited substances since most animals are injected that makes them grow faster

- Less chance of getting sick before an important test (as happened in Club de Cuervos)

- Satisfaction for performing better while helping to take care of our planet

PatrikBaboumian (the current strongest man in the world) mentions in The Game Changers that "sometimes someone asked me how can you be as strong as a Bull if you don't eat meat ?, to which I replied, **have you ever seen a Bull eat meat?"**

Take care of your body and the planet.

10 Most Delicious and Easy-Peasy Plant-based Recipes from my Kitchen

Cooking healthy, rich, and fast is possible, and to show you that it is true, I want to share these 15 easy vegan recipes that are ready in less than 30 minutes.

They are very simple recipes, both sweet and savory, and among which you will find breakfasts, snacks, desserts, lunches, and dinners.

In general, I tried to keep the recipes simple and have less than ten ingredients or that you need less than 30 minutes to prepare them. In this compilation, you can find some of my favorites.

If there is an ingredient that you do not like or cannot find, read the complete entry because I usually give different options. If not, you can modify the recipe without a problem or ask by leaving a comment. Our recipes are generally easy to adapt and give a lot of play, so I encourage you to prepare them for your liking, using the ingredients you usually have in your kitchen.

1. Vegan chocolate pudding: To make this chocolate pudding, you only need five ingredients, and it is ready in 5 minutes. You can add the toppings that you like the most. I have added coconut whipped cream and caramel syrup.

You only need five ingredients and 5 minutes to prepare this vegan chocolate pudding. You can add your favorite toppings.

- **Preparation:** 5 mins
- **Total:** 5 mins
- **Servings:** 2
- **Category:** Sweet
- **Cuisine:** Vegan, Gluten-Free

INGREDIENTS

- 1/4 cup of rice milk (62g)
- 1/2 cup of unsweetened cocoa powder (50g)
- 1/2 cup of maple syrup (180g)
- 1 banana
- 1 avocado
- 1 teaspoon vanilla extract (optional)
- Toppings: coconut whipped cream and caramel syrup

INSTRUCTIONS

1. Put all the ingredients in a food processor, food processor, or mixer and beat until you get the desired consistency.

2. Serve the pudding in individual cups or containers. You can eat it fresh, but it is richer if you wait at least 2 hours or even overnight.

3. Scoop the toppings just before serving.

2. Spinach with chickpeas: This dish is very typical of Seville, and although it is very simple, it is one of my favorite ways of eating chickpeas. This version is lighter because it has less oil.

Spinach with chickpeas is a typical dish of Spanish cuisine. It is a simple but very tasty recipe. Besides, this version is lighter.

- **Preparation:** 5 mins
- **Cook:** 15 mins
- **Total:** 20 minutes
- **Servings:** 4
- **Category:** Chickpeas
- **Cuisine:** Vegan, Gluten-Free

INGREDIENTS

- Extra virgin olive oil
- 1 head of garlic (12 cloves)
- 3 tablespoons of sweet paprika
- 6 cups of spinach (250 g)
- 1/2 cup of water (125 ml)
- 3 and 1/2 cups of cooked chickpeas (650 g)
- Salt (optional)

INSTRUCTIONS

1. In a frying pan, add a splash of oil, and when it is hot, add the chopped garlic. Cook them over medium heat until golden brown.

2. Add the paprika, stir and add the chopped spinach. You can add plenty of oil to cook the spinach or use 1/2 cup of water. Leave the spinach for about 5 minutes. You can also add salt, although I do not add it.

3. Add the chickpeas, stir, and if you want, you can add a little more paprika or oil—Cook for about 5 more minutes.

3. Zucchini spaghetti with avocado sauce: This zucchini spaghetti is lighter and healthier than conventional spaghetti. This recipe is ideal if you want something fast and healthy, which also nourishes your body and makes you feel great.

This recipe for zucchini spaghetti with avocado sauce is prepared in less than 10 minutes. It is light, healthy, and very nutritious.

- **Preparation:** 10 mins
- **Total:** 10 mins
- **Servings:** 2
- **Category:** Pasta
- **Cuisine:** Vegan, Raw Vegan, Gluten-Free

INGREDIENTS

- 1 zucchini
- 1/3 cup of water (85 ml)
- 2 tablespoons lemon juice
- 1 avocado
- 4 tablespoons pine nuts
- 1 1/4 cup of fresh basil (30 g)
- 12 cherry tomatoes

INSTRUCTIONS

1. Make the zucchini pasta.
2. Beat the rest of the ingredients except the tomatoes in a mixer or food processor.
3. Put the pasta in a bowl, add the sauce, mix well, and add the tomatoes.

4. Chocolate oatmeal porridge: Oatmeal porridge is the ideal breakfast, especially when it's cold. This version has chocolate and coconut milk. You can use any non-dairy milk if you don't like coconut milk and add your favorite fruits.

This chocolate oatmeal porridge is ready in 15 minutes, and you only need 5 ingredients. They are ideal to have a rich and healthy breakfast.

- **Preparation:** 5 mins
- **Cook:** 10 mins

- **Total:** 15 minutes
- **Servings:** 2
- **Category:** Sweet
- **Cuisine:** Vegan

INGREDIENTS

- 1 1/2 cups of coconut milk (375 ml)
- 1/2 cup of water (125 ml)
- 1/2 cup of rolled oats (80 g)
- 4 tablespoons unsweetened cocoa powder
- 8 tablespoons coconut sugar
- Toppings: strawberries, chocolate chips, and grated coconut to taste

INSTRUCTIONS

1. Pour the coconut milk and water into a saucepan and turn the heat to high. When it's hot (but before it comes to a boil), turn down to medium or medium-high heat and add the oats. Cover the saucepan and cook for 5 to 10 minutes or until the oatmeal is done.

2. Take the saucepan off the heat and add the cocoa and sugar. Stir until they dissolve, and all the ingredients are well integrated.

3. Serve the porridge in a bowl and add your favorite toppings.

5. Vegan miso soup: I love to eat this soup at dinner time. It is very comforting and is ready in less than 15 minutes. You only need 6 ingredients to prepare it, and it is also very tasty.

This vegan miso soup is prepared in 15 minutes. It is light, healthy, tasty, and very comforting. It is the perfect dinner!

- **Preparation:** 10 mins
- **Cook:** 5 mins
- **Total:** 15 minutes
- **Servings:** 3
- **Category:** Soup
- **Cuisine:** Vegan, Japanese

INGREDIENTS

- 40 g noodles
- 3 tablespoons miso
- 1 liter of water
- 1 tablespoon wakame seaweed
- 100 g soft tofu
- 1/2 cup of chives (60 g)

INSTRUCTIONS

1. Cook the noodles or the type of pasta you use following the instructions on the package.

2. Put the miso in a bowl.

3. Pour the water into a pot, and when it comes to a boil, add a little water to the bowl in which you had the miso. Stir until dissolved.

4. Add the wakame seaweed to the pot and cook over medium-high heat for about 5 minutes.

5. Remove the pot from the heat, add the mixture of water and miso that you had in the bowl, the chopped tofu, and the spring onion, and stir. If you want, you can cook the tofu and chives a little, although it is not necessary. Remember that miso should not be heated because if not, it loses its properties.

6. Add the already cooked noodles last.

6. Vegan fat-free macaroni and cheese: Pasta has a very bad reputation, but if you use healthy ingredients, you can include it in your regular diet without fear of getting fat. This sauce is similar to our vegan cheese, but it is fat-free.

These Fat-Free Vegan Mac n Cheese are so light and rich. You can use the cheese sauce to prepare other recipes or as a dip.

- **Preparation:** 5 mins
- **Cook:** 15 mins
- **Total:** 20 minutes
- **Servings:** 4
- **Category:** Pasta
- **Cuisine:** Vegan, Gluten-Free

INGREDIENTS

- 240 g gluten-free pasta (8.5 oz)
- 2 and 1/2 cups of cauliflower (450 g)
- 1/2 cup of water (125 ml)
- 2 teaspoons garlic powder
- 2 teaspoons onion powder
- 1/4 cup of nutritional yeast or brewer's yeast (16 g)
- 1 tablespoon of lemon juice
- 2 tablespoons soy sauce
- 1/4 teaspoon turmeric

INSTRUCTIONS

1. Cook the pasta according to the instructions on the package.
2. Meanwhile, steam the cauliflower or in plenty of boiling water until tender (about 10-15 minutes).
3. Add the cauliflower to a blender with the rest of the ingredients and beat until they are perfectly integrated. Add salt if it seems bland.
4. Mix the pasta with the sauce in a pot or pan or directly on the plate.

7. Smoothie bowl: This recipe is a different way to enjoy the famous fruit and vegetable smoothies or smoothies. Children love it because it has a delicious chocolate flavor and is also very healthy and nutritious.

Smoothie bowl, a different way of drinking smoothies, which is also easier to digest. You only need 3 ingredients and 5 minutes to prepare it.

- **Preparation:** 5 mins
- **Total:** 5 mins
- **Servings:** 2
- **Category:** Breakfast
- **Cuisine:** American, Vegan

INGREDIENTS

- 2 bananas, frozen
- 1 cup of frozen blueberries (140 g)

- 1 cup of vegetable milk or water (250 ml), I used oat milk unsweetened
- 2 tablespoons peanut butter, optional
- 2 Medjool dates, optional

INSTRUCTIONS

1. Put all the ingredients in a powerful mixer and beat until well combined.
2. Serve in a bowl and decorate with your favorite toppings (I added fresh blueberries and chopped almonds, and pistachios).
3. The ideal is to take it fresh, but you can keep it in an airtight container in the fridge for 1 or 2 days.

8.Vegan Greek salad: It is a very fresh and easy to make the salad. I have prepared my own vegan Feta cheese, much lighter, cholesterol-free, and just as rich as the original.

Vegan Greek salad with Feta tofu cheese. A very light, healthy, and nutritious salad. It is delicious and only has 202 calories per serving.

- **Preparation:** 10 mins
- **Total:** 10 mins
- **Servings:** 4
- **Category:** Salad
- **Cuisine:** Vegan, Gluten-Free

INGREDIENTS

- 1/2 red onion
- 1 cucumber
- 1 green pepper
- 4 tomatoes
- Vegan Feta Cheese
- 40 black olives
- 1 tablespoon of oregano
- Extra virgin olive oil
- Salt and black pepper to taste (optional)

INSTRUCTIONS

1. Chop the vegetables, add the vegan Feta cheese and the dressing. We mix well, and we have our salad ready.

9. Three delicious vegan rice: This rice is ideal if you don't want to complicate your life a lot but want a satisfying and tasty dish. You can add soy sauce, tamari, sweet and sour sauce, or whatever sauce you like best.

The three delicious vegan rice is prepared in about 15 or 20 minutes. It is a quick, simple, healthy, light, inexpensive, and delicious dish.

- **Preparation:** 5 mins
- **Cook:** 15 mins
- **Total:** 20 minutes
- **Servings:** 2
- **Category:** Rice
- **Cuisine:** Vegan, Gluten-Free

INGREDIENTS

- 3/4 cup of rice (150 g)
- Extra virgin olive oil
- 1 carrot
- 1/4 cup frozen peas (35 g)
- 75 g tofu (2.7 ounces)
- 1/8 teaspoon turmeric
- Sea salt (optional)
- 1 tablespoon soy sauce or tamari

INSTRUCTIONS

1. Cook the rice according to the manufacturer's instructions and let it cool. Ideally, you should cook it the day before. If you are in a hurry, you can cool the rice with cold water.

2. In a frying pan, add a little oil and fry the finely chopped carrot for about 2 minutes. Add the peas and cook for about 3 more minutes. Put them on a plate.

3. Chop the tofu and mash it with a fork until it looks similar to scrambled eggs.

4. Pour a little more oil into the pan and sauté the tofu with the turmeric and a little salt (optional) for about 5 minutes. Put it on the plate where you had the vegetables.

5. Add a splash of oil again and sauté the rice for about 2 minutes. Add the vegetables, tofu, soy sauce, or tamari and cook for 3 more minutes.

10. Vegan apple custard: If you like apples, you have to try these custards. The recipe is incredibly simple, and the result is spectacular.

These vegan apple custards are ready in about 15 or 20 minutes and are the perfect dessert. They are healthy, delicious, and very easy to prepare.

- **Preparation:** 5 mins
- **Cook:** 15 mins
- **Total:** 20 minutes
- **Servings:** 4
- **Category:** Sweet
- **Cuisine:** Vegan

INGREDIENTS

- 2 apples
- The juice of half a lemon
- 4 tablespoons agave syrup or coconut sugar
- 4 cups of oat milk (1 liter)
- 1 piece of a vanilla bean (about 1 inch or 2 centimeters)
- 1 large or 2 small cinnamon sticks
- 1 or 2 teaspoons of agar powder

INSTRUCTIONS

1. Peel the apples and chop them.
2. In a saucepan, add the apples, lemon juice, agave syrup, or coconut sugar (or whatever sweetener you want). Cook for about 5 minutes so that the apple falls apart and softens.
3. Add the milk, vanilla, and cinnamon, and turn the heat to the highest. When it comes to a boil, lower the heat and cook for about 5 minutes.
4. Add the agar powder and cook for another 5 minutes.
5. Remove the cinnamon stick, beat the custard, and serve in individual bowls. If you do not have a perfect texture when cooling, you can beat them again before serving.

The growth factors of meat and their impact on health

The word bacteria is known all over the world and is usually associated with the disease. What few people know is the **new name "superbug. "** Superbugs or growth factors that are applied to animals that serve us as food are not known and have a lot to do with our health.

What are superbugs?

So far, **antibiotics** were seen as a way to fight various infectious diseases. Unfortunately, these drugs are losing their positive side and evolving to represent one of the greatest **threats to the health** of all the inhabitants of the planet: superbugs.

Superbug is the term used when talking about **strains of bacteria resistant to most of the antibiotics** that we use regularly.

According to a report on antibiotic resistance carried out by the British Government: *"if urgent measures are not put in place, in the year 2050 more people could die from superbugs than from cancer or traffic accidents".*

The **use and abuse** of these drugs have led many people to develop **resistance to antibiotics**. Microbes, over time, have managed to become healthy. However, this is not the only reason why bacteria have turned into superbugs. **The meat of the animals** that we bring to our table also has a lot to do with it.

Animals for human consumption

Another cause of the existence of superbugs is **the farms of animals destined for** human **consumption**. Be it pigs, cows, or chickens, **any of these animals spend their entire lives receiving antibiotic treatments**. The reason is not only the treatment of diseases but also the **prevention and breeding elements**, for example, **for fattening**. As is logical, the more they are consumed, the more excellent the resistance.

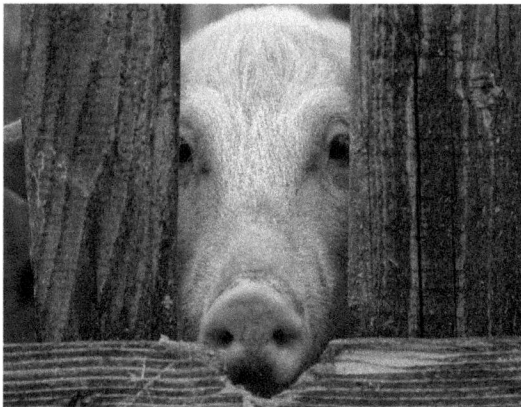

According to James Tiedje, professor of Microbiology and Molecular Genetics at the University of Michigan: "These resistant bacteria also transmit their resistance and defense mechanisms to other microorganisms in the environment and man."

These animals, besides, are subjected to a type of life that makes them susceptible to all kinds of diseases. For example, a chicken that would need 52 weeks to weigh 4kg in these farms will have to do it in just 12 weeks. They are fooled by altering the light cycles or keeping the light on all day. They are also not allowed to move so that they do not waste calories, and the use of antibiotics is massive.

For their part, it is widespread for shepherds to sell their calves or reeds to intermediaries. These will see to it that these animals get fat and grow at full speed, whatever the cost. The critical thing is profitability. Here the dignity and health of the animal are not respected, and the health of future consumers.

Measures are taken but not in all countries

To avoid these problems, some countries like the US proposed an initiative to avoid that, as up to now, 70% of the antibiotics supplied in that country were for animals destined for human consumption. In turn, the European Union joined the proposal made by the World Health Organization, and, in 2006, the ban on this type of drug for the growth of animals was agreed upon.

Unfortunately, there are other countries where antibiotics for animals are poorly or poorly regulated. One such country is China, where antibiotics are used routinely on farms.

Bovine growth hormones

In addition to antibiotics, other types of substances are also used that contribute to the fattening of cattle. The Hormone Recombinant Growth Bovin (rBGH) or Somatotropin is a hormone obtained by genetic engineering, which copies the hormone cows produce naturally. This hormone is designed so that cows produce more milk than they would typically produce. Its mission is to alter the gene expression for glucose transporters in the cow's mammary gland, muscle, and fat. This gene makes the transfer of glucose to the mammary gland easier, leading to higher milk production.

How could it be otherwise? These treatments are not without problems and side effects. The danger of its use is such that its use is prohibited in the European Union and Canada. Still, in some countries like the US, it has been used for several years.

The economic benefit of the extra amount of milk that the cow can offer does not benefit the animal. Animals that are treated with this hormone suffer great stress. Only after 12 weeks after the cow is a calf will it begin to produce milk, although its health suffers. During the treatment, you will lose weight, you will stop being fertile, and you will be very susceptible to all kinds of diseases. At a certain point, milk production decreases, and the cow's body begins to recover. At that time, the rBGH is injected, and the farmer postpones that recovery for another 8 or 12 weeks. As is customary, the increase in milk production will be directly proportional to the risk of disease to which the animal is subjected.

The problem happens to the milk

The biggest problem with this treatment is the increased risk of mastitis. The cow that suffers from mastitis produces milk with pus. This could be a cause of the rejection of milk by dairy companies. What solution will farmers find to avoid losing income? Antibiotics again!

Again, antibiotics will be used to cure mastitis in cows. This would not be necessary if economic profitability were not above the welfare of animals and people.

We are putting our lives in danger by trying to manipulate nature. Human sensitivity should always be ahead of economic profitability.

Chapter 4: Sugar, the real culprit, and why are vegans concerned about B12

When we talk about sugar consumption, we must bear in mind that **75% of what we eat comes from products such as cookies, soft drinks, or packaged sauces**. Although we need glucose to live, it is no secret that the excess amount of sugar found in some **everyday foods** can take its toll.

The World Health Organization (WHO) recommended in 2003 not to exceed 10% of our energy intake of free sugars, which are those added to food during manufacture and preparation and sugars naturally present in foods such as fruits or honey. This means that an adult person with a body mass index (BMI) between 18.5 and 25 can consume **about twelve sugar cubes a day** or, what is the same, 48 grams a day.

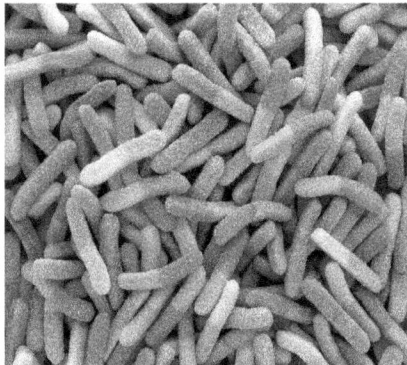

However, several countries in the European Union recommend consuming a maximum **of 25 grams of free sugar per day** (or 5% of the total energy), about six small tablespoons. However, according to data from the European Food Safety Authority (EFSA), we could consume between

16% and 36% more. What happens when we overeat sugar? What signals does the body send us to tell us that we are passing?

The five signs of excess sugar

Consuming too much sugar puts our bodies on alert in several ways. These are the five ways in which it can affect our body:

1. Caries

When we consume sugar, oral bacteria become more active, multiplying and forming plaque on the teeth' surface. This sticky film produces an acid that dissolves the minerals that cover the outside of the tooth.

This process results in the formation of small holes or an increase in the tooth's porosity until cavities appear. It can also happen that this bacterial plaque settles on the gums and turns into gingivitis.

2. Obesity

Sugar turns into glucose when it reaches the body. When we eat too much, the pancreas' insulin and its function keep blood sugar levels stable and transfer excess sugar to the cells.

Research published in the *American Journal of Clinical Nutrition* in 2011 confirmed a positive association between regular consumption of soft drinks and the growing epidemic of obesity. In people with a sedentary life, only a small part already serves as an energy store, and most of it will be transformed into fat stores.

3. Skin problems

Sugar leads to increased sebum production and can promote skin problems, such as acne or eczema. In a **study** with 2,300 adolescents, it was shown, for example, that those who consume more added sugar have a 30% higher risk of developing acne.

Other research has linked excess sugar to difficulty in repairing collagen, the protein that maintains the skin. An excessively sweet diet can reduce elasticity and promote the appearance of premature wrinkles.

4. The body asks for more

"I need something sweet" is a common phrase that who else has heard or said the least. When we eat sugar, the pancreas secretes insulin, which allows the sugar to penetrate the cells and promotes the penetration of L-tryptophan into the brain, an amino acid used in serotonin production. This neurotransmitter creates a feeling of wellbeing.

Research published in Neuroscience& *Biobehavioral Reviews* noted in 2008 that when given to rats unlimited access to sugar, these had four signs of addiction: bingeing, withdrawal, anxiety, and a possible gateway to other substances.

The study concluded that sugar could be addictive only when consumed compulsively. Another thing is that when we feel down or discouraged, the body tries to raise this "hormone of happiness" by giving it a dose of sugar.

5. Fatigue and tiredness

Lack of energy is a sign that there is too much sugar in the blood. Although foods high in added sugar quickly increase blood sugar and insulin levels, leading to increased energy, this is fleeting and temporary because it plummets.

Sugar-laden products lack protein, fiber, or fat, leading to a brief surge in energy, followed by a sharp drop in blood sugar. Also, in most cases, foods high in sugar crowd out whole grains and contribute to **nutritional deficiencies**, according to the American Heart Association (AHA).

Alternatives to sugar
The prevention of all these signs goes through moderation. Foods that naturally contain sugar generally also contain fiber, vitamins, minerals, and water. Fruits and some vegetables are good examples of foods that we should be consuming more of.

Ghost sugar: ten foods that have it and you don't suspect it

Ghost sugar is **that hidden ingredient that you cannot see in a food product** but is often disproportionately present. It can be compared to added sugar, but many times it is not the same because ghost sugar sometimes belongs intrinsically to the food's nature and therefore does not need to be added.

Other times, it is the sugar that has been introduced to enhance the appetite for sweet taste or to cover certain bad smells, textures, or deficiencies. In all cases, it is a sugar that we do not suspect is there, and that many times we cannot identify when tasting the food. And yet it is there.

Beyond sugary drinks

The presence of sugar in all types of carbonated soft drinks is notable and known, as well as in most **cakes and biscuits, in sweets of all kinds, breakfast cereals**, etc. We are aware of its amount of sugar, and based on this, we can avoid or moderate its consumption, which is harmful to our cardiovascular health.

However, in the case of ghost sugar, by definition, we are **unaware of its existence** in products that seem perfectly normal to us and that we eat without awareness of its destructive potential. That is why it is convenient to know them to moderate their consumption or opt for healthier ones. Here we explain ten of these foods with ghost sugar.

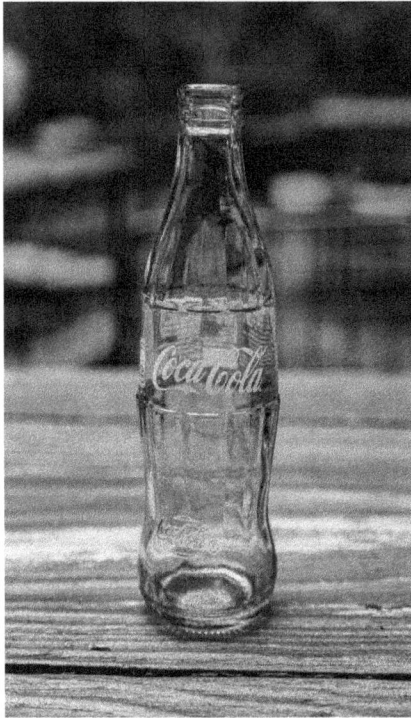

The 'dirty ten' of ghost sugar

1. Sliced bread

A medium sliced bread contains approximately 8 to 10 grams of sugar for every two slices, which means that there are between 16 and 20 grams in a pair of sandwiches, the equivalent of three lumps.

2. Industrial sauces

From the ubiquitous ketchup to canned tomato sauces, to all kinds of mustards and salad vinaigrettes, the presence of sugar is significant, reaching an average of 21 grams per 100 grams of sauce. Usually, the sweet taste is hidden behind more robust flavors such as sour – as in some Modena vinegar – or salty, but it exerts its harmful influence on health.

3. Pizzas

Do not forget that the pizzas are made with refined flour dough, which is nothing more than pure and hard starch, broken down into glucose in the intestine. Therefore, the pizza base releases large amounts of ghost sugar that can be avoided **if the pizza is made with whole wheat flour**, something scarce.

4. Diet bars

Many people consume **these types of bars** as a supplement after sports or as a substitute for a regular meal. These people do not know that this type of product can carry **up to 36 grams of sugar per 100 of product.**

The composition is usually specified in an elusive way: they contain sugar, glucose syrup, sugar from the raisins they carry, dextrose - another name for glucose - and invert sugar syrup: the trick of **calling sugar its 56 different names.**

5. Fruit juice

Natural **fruit juices** already have a remarkable amount of intrinsic sugar. Still, if we go to industrial packaged and concentrated juices, we will see that **these glucose levels skyrocket** many times.

According to a study **published in 2016 in the Journal of Nutrition** and based on people with cardiovascular risk, drinking more than five glasses per week of sugary or sweetened beverages, including diet drinks and fruit juices, increases abdominal obesity, hypertension blood triglyceride levels and lowers good cholesterol.

6. Light yogurts

Another case is that of **myths about light foods**, such as yogurt. One of them is that they lose weight because they provide fewer calories. It is false since the method to measure them is based on the fats in milk, when what is truly harmful are the added sugars that they often present. Although some yogurt without added sugar, it is practically impossible to find it in the light range.

7. Industrial spreadable cheeses

Another classic example of ghost sugars is melted cheese spreads, which have little to do with what we usually understand by cheese.

8. Some vegetable 'milk'

Within the range of vegetable drinks, we must be careful when selecting them for our consumption since many of them include not a few added sugars, as can be read in their nutritional composition. We will always select those whose percentage does not exceed 6-7%.

9. Sushi

We come to sushi and, therefore, to the great problem of refined rice, that is, without dietary fiber. The same thing happens with pizza: rice, like wheat, is a cereal, and cereals accumulate starch in their seeds, that is, long chains of sugars. The recommendation is not to abuse these types of dishes.

10. Chocolate

Dark chocolate is a mass of cocoa paste with sugar, and the percentage of this ingredient can vary from 50% to 1% in the case of chocolates with 99% cocoa, which would be the only recommended ones.

If we talk about milk chocolate, the sugar shoots up in this product, as it results from the mixture of cocoa butter, rich in sugars, with condensed milk. A product, therefore really harmful.

Vitamin B12: why you have a problem if you are vegan

What exactly is vitamin B12? What is it for, and what does it mean? Vitamin B12 deficiency? Is it true that it is exclusively of animal origin? Is it true that a vegetarian diet needs to be supplemented with vitamin B12? Is there no plant-based vitamin B12?

People ask me a **few questions, and all of them interesting**, so we will answer them one by one to unravel the problems that revolve around the achievement of this vitamin in certain dietary philosophies such as vegetarians and vegans. Let's start with the first one.

What exactly is vitamin B12?

Vitamin **B12** or **cobalamin** is one of the vitamins with a more complex structure. It consists of several amino compounds and aromatic (denominated vitamers) that relate to each other by a cobalt ion, which maintains its spatial structure. It is a water-soluble vitamin essential for the brain's normal functioning, the nervous system, and the formation of blood and different proteins.

On the other hand, it is generally **involved in the metabolism of the human body's cells**, especially in the synthesis and regulation of DNA and the metabolization of amino acids, fatty acids, and carbohydrates. In other words, it is essential for the proper functioning of the digestive process and the assimilation of food, as well as for neurological development and cell division.

What is vitamin B12 deficiency for, and what does it mean?

It is a compound that we cannot live without; hence it is called a vitamin. Its absence or deficit in our body can have various consequences. The most obvious symptom is the so-called **pernicious anemia**, a condition in which the body does not have enough red blood cells and cannot correctly supply oxygen to the body tissues.

Symptoms are shortness of breath, fatigue, paleness, high heart rate, lack of appetite, diarrhea, numbness of the hands and feet with a tingling sensation, or mouth ulcers, among some others. They may be because **our intestines do not want to fix and absorb vitamin B12** or because this, in its active form, is not present in our diet in sufficient quantities. If the deficit persists for a long time, it can lead to chronic depression or even have more serious neurological consequences.

Is it true that it is of exclusively animal origin?

Vitamin B12 **is not of animal origin**, but it is true that until now, it has been found that, with some exceptions such as nori seaweed, humans can only get it in its active form from meats - mammals, poultry, fish, and some seafood-, eggs-raw- and dairy products. That is, only from animal and non-vegetable sources, at least in sufficient quantities.

Now, the only real producers of cyanocobalamin and its analogous forms -which resemble it but are not active for our metabolism-, are **some groups of bacteria and Archea**, unicellular beings previously located in the prokaryotic kingdom. Each animal then obtains it from this source in its way, either from the environment or from bacteria that nest in its intestinal flora or the rumen, as is the case with ruminants.

But humans **can only get it from animal sources**, given the confirmation of our intestinal flora, our type of diet, and the access we have to previously washed vegetables, which eliminate the possible bacteria that manufacture B12.

Is it true that a vegetarian diet needs to be supplemented with vitamin B12?

Recently I contacted several **nutritionists of reference in vegan issues**, and he explains the problems that the obtaining of cyanocobalamin from plant sources implies for a strict vegetarian. In the case of non-strict vegetarians who consume, for example, dairy products such as cheese or yogurt, does not have to be a problem.

All-vegan people should supplement with vitamin B12 from various sources, either with enriched foods or directly with daily and weekly supplements, preferably with the semi-synthetic form known as **cyanocobalamin**, a modification from the compound original generated by bacteria cultures.

In this regard, all vitamin B12 supplements are **manufactured from bacterial sources**, and none contemplate animal exploitation to obtain it.

Isn't there a vitamin B12 of plant origin?

It exists in certain groups of algae, brewer's yeast, and in a few vegetables. Still, with very few exceptions, these **do not contain the effective version for human metabolism but rather an analogous one**, useful for bacteria but does not work in our physiology. The same is true for mussels, a source highly recommended so far.

Also, ingesting these B12-like compounds can be counterproductive because they **can interfere with the proteins responsible for binding cobalamin** and carrying it to cells. That is why supplementation with enriched foods in addition to weekly or daily pills is recommended for vegans. Additionally, a tea ferment called **kombucha** could be a source of active B12, but there are no conclusive studies.

B12: absorption, types, and supplementation

This is the third post in the series on B12 in vegetarians. In case you have missed the first two, I leave them here:

Absorption of V12

The B12 contained in food is bound to proteins. The action of hydrochloric acid and pepsin (an enzyme that hydrolyzes proteins) in the stomach cause B12 to separate from those proteins to which it is attached and bind to other proteins called cobalophilin B12-binding proteins. They are released in turn when pancreatic proteases act. At that time, if PH conditions are favorable, it binds to intrinsic factor (IF), forming a complex that is recognized by specific receptors in the terminal ileum (a part of the intestine thin) where it is absorbed. Inside the intestine cells, it passes into TC2, which we had already mentioned was the protein that was responsible for transporting B12 through the body.

This happens when we talk about physiological doses, which are the amounts of B12 in food or even in daily supplementation. But let's talk about pharmacological doses (1000mcg or more). Absorption no longer depends on FI, and B12 can spread across the intestinal barrier, appearing in the blood much earlier than by the previous route, which can be used in individuals with absorption problems, avoiding having to inject B12 since supplementation at pharmacological doses has proven to be just as effective, even in gastrectomy patients.

We know that there is a reserve of B12 that is mainly found in the liver. Besides, the body reuses part of the B12 through the enterohepatic route and other compounds such as cholesterol. This means that a part of the B12 is salvaged for reuse instead of being expelled in the feces. These two factors (existing reserve and enterohepatic recovery) mean that the B12 deficit may take years to manifest (up to 4 years, most sources coincide).

But beware, this does NOT mean that anyone's reserves last four years, but that some people can last about four years. It may take you one. It is impossible to know since we do not generally know the previous state of these reserves, nor is the enterohepatic recovery equally efficient in all people and depends on other factors.

Therefore, the recommendation is to supplement B12 from the moment you start a vegetarian diet, not deplete the reserve and prevent a deficit. It is important to bear in mind that once the reserve is depleted, the drop is steep. We have already commented on the difficulties in diagnosing the deficit in vegetarians in previous posts.

Vitamin B12 types

- **Methylcobalamin:** is the form in which B12 is in the blood and also in some foods

- **5-deoxyadenosylcobalamin:** (may also be called dibencozide or adenosylcobalamin) is the way B12 is stored in the liver
- **Cyanocobalamin:** is one of the common forms in supplements and fortified foods
- **Hydroxycobalamin: it** is the most common form in food

Although methylcobalamin and dibeconzide offer absorption benefits, supplementation with cyanocobalamin is recommended for several reasons:

- It is the most stable form, and best resists temperature, light, and variations in PH.
- It is the cheapest presentation and the easiest to find, and we are talking about long-term supplementation.
- It is the most studied form as a supplement. We can say that it is safe even at absurdly high doses, while other forms of B12 have not been sufficiently studied to recommend its use as a long-term supplement. Both the US Institute of Medicine and the UK Expert Group on Vitamins and Minerals impact its safety. Not even a maximum dose is set. Likewise, experts in vegetarian nutrition such as Norris, Mangels, and Messina recommend that B12 supplementation be done with cyanocobalamin because there is also not enough research to establish long-term supplementation doses in the other forms of B12 supplementation with methylcobalamin should be at higher doses than cyanocobalamin, so if someone uses the recommended doses for cyanocobalamin in methylcobalamin, they may not get adequate supplementation.

However, in cases of an established deficit, pathologies, or special situations, it may be advisable to use methylcobalamin or dibeconzide in a specific or long-term manner in specific patients. But that must be assessed individually by a professional. In principle, in healthy vegetarians, the recommendation is to use cyanocobalamin.

Likewise, it should be noted that smokers excrete more cyanocobalamin because their cyanide levels are high, so vegan smokers whose only source of B12 was cyanocobalamin could present a greater risk of deficiency due to a high excretion of it. This is a hypothesis because there are no studies on smoking vegans. Norris suggests that it would be prudent to supplement this case withmethylcobalamin (500-1000mcg/day) but continue to give cyanocobalamin doses for greater safety.

Recommended supplementation dose for healthy adults

We have three options, taking into account that they are not aimed at people with an established deficit, but what are maintenance options:
- Take daily foods enriched in B12 (enriched vegetable drinks, enriched soy yogurts, enriched cereals), making sure to reach 2.4 mcg daily in two doses.
- Take a daily supplement of 25-100mcg. If it is in a pill, it must be chewed since saliva provides Haptocorrin that favors absorption.
- Take a weekly supplement of 2000mcg or one of 1000mcg twice a week. In this case, it can be swallowed without chewing since it is considered a pharmacological dose and directly diffuses the enteric barrier, as we have commented.

The percentage of absorption of B12 depends on the size of the dose. Therefore, they do not follow a mathematical correlation. The higher the dose, the lower the absorption percentage.

There are already many products enriched with B12 in Spain, the most common being some vegetable drinks and some breakfast cereals, but in my opinion, they are not a good option, let me explain:

To name some well-known and nationally available products, vegetable drinks (soy and almond, not oatmeal) provide 0.38mcg of B12 in a glass (250ml), so it would be necessary to consume a high daily amount of the product to meet requirements, which is not advisable within the framework of a healthy diet.

On the other hand, the corn flakes breakfast cereals provide 0.63mcg of B12 per 30g serving, which leaves us in a situation similar to the previous one. And I have taken the corn flakes as the example because they are the ones with the least sugar...

In addition to these two examples of well-known products, there are many options for enriched products from different brands. It is necessary to consult the nutritional labeling carefully if you want to meet the requirements of B12 based on these foods and take into account that it can not be the most suitable option since it is also by definition highly processed products rich in sugar, despite being the most similar way to the natural contribution in food.

In a healthy adult, I would opt for 2000mcg per week, which is the most comfortable supplementation, which comes at the best price, and which also has guaranteed absorption in cases of hypochlorhydria.

Where to get the daily dose of B12?

In recent years, the vegetarian eating style has increased in popularity. The decision can be for ethical and ecological reasons, but also health reasons. In some cases, certain nutritional aspects of such a choice may be unknown, which can lead to disorders that alter serum glucose, blood pressure, or body mass.

The fact that following a diet of this type, if not done in a balanced and correct way, should not be underestimated, can lead to nutritional deficiencies due to the absence of certain nutrients. As the American Dietetic Association (ADA) recognizes, doing it properly, in a planned way, and under the supervision of a nutritionist is healthy and can provide benefits. There is an important aspect of concern if it is not done well, and special attention should be paid: vitamin B12.

What happens if we don't get enough vitamin B12?

Vitamin B12, also called cobalamin because it contains cobalt ore, is soluble in water and is found in significant amounts in animal origin foods such as fish, meat, poultry, eggs, and milk, but little presence in the vegetable. It should be specified that vitamin B12 comes from the synthesis of microorganisms ingested by animals.

Some types of B12 are:

- Methylcobalamin and 5-deoxyadenosylcabobalamin are the forms of vitamin B12 active in human metabolism and offer absorption benefits.
- Cyanocobalamin, one of the most common forms in fortified foods.
- Hydroxycobalamin, which is the most common in food.

The amount of vitamin B12 is important, especially in meat and fish and, to a lesser extent, in other foods such as:

- Cooked eggs: 0.6 mcg per 50 grams.
- 100 grams of whole milk, 0.3 mcg; semi-skimmed milk, 0.4 mcg; skim milk, 0.22mcg.
- A natural yogurt: 0.37 mcg.
- 100 grams of fresh cheese: 0.66 mcg.

This vitamin is necessary to properly form red blood cells, neurological function, and DNA synthesis. The recommendations for vitamin B12 intake from the European Food Safety Authority (EFSA) are:
- 4 micrograms (µg) a day for those over 15 years of age.
- 4.5 µg for pregnant women.
- 5 µg for nursing mothers.

Suppose the consumption of products of animal origin is low or null. In that case, there may be a deficiency that translates, in some cases, into weight loss, fatigue, weakness, constipation, loss of appetite and weight, and anemia. Neurological changes such as numbness and tingling in the hands and feet can also occur.

How to get the necessary vitamin B12?

People who follow a vegetarian diet have to be careful because plant origin foods do not contain sufficient amounts in an active form. Among vegetarians, the strictest, those who do not consume eggs or dairy products, have the highest risk. Where can you find this source of the vitamin if you are vegan or vegan?

The fortified cereals for breakfast can be a ready source of highly bioavailable vitamin B12 for vegetarians, and some nutritional products enriched yeast. These are some of the few vitamin B12 from plants and can be used as dietary sources for strict vegetarians. But, despite all this, a vegetarian person will hardly reach the daily recommendations.

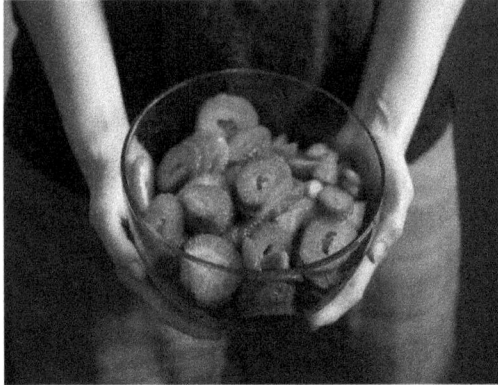

It should also be taken into account that other foods of plant origin that are associated as a source of B12 (spirulina algae, brewer's yeast, or fermented algae) do not contain B12 in its active form, but rather that they have analogs known as corrinoids, insufficient to meet the needs of metabolism. These corrinoids can also mask a possible deficiency of the vitamin in a blood test if algae consumption is abused, recognizes the Spanish Society of Diet and Food Sciences (SEDCA).

The importance of supplements

Therefore, both vegetarians should supplement their diet with vitamin B12 to avoid the risk of long-term deficiency. Supplementation is important to reach the B12 recommendations. They would have to consume very high amounts of eggs, milk, or dairy products every day (about seven eggs a day or about four glasses of milk).

It is known, due to the peculiarities of this vitamin, which is found mainly in the liver, the body has a reserve of B12 that it can reuse instead of excreting it in the feces. This means that the deficiency can take months, even years, to manifest. For this reason, it is advisable, when starting a vegetarian diet, to supplement B12 in order not to deplete the reserves in the body prematurely and thus prevent the deficit.

For supplementation, it is recommended that B12 is in the form of cyanocobalamin, considered the most stable to light, changes in pH, temperature and does not have a toxic dose. The nutritionist is the one who must assess what, how, and how much should be taken as a supplement to reach the recommended daily micrograms (it can be worth a daily or weekly supplement).

Chapter 5: The Microbiome Diet

With the microbiome diet, you can take care of your intestinal flora, but not only. A healthy microbiome can also help you get in shape and lose weight. But to get the best results, you shouldn't just focus on what you eat: physical activity, good rest, and a stress-free life also help you improve the characteristics of the population of microbes living in your intestine.

When it comes to losing weight, the wellbeing of the intestinal flora can be crucial. For this reason, if you want to lose weight, you could find the solution for you in the microbiome diet, a diet not specifically designed to eliminate excess pounds but which can have weight loss as a welcome side effect.

Its main purpose is to promote a good balance of the intestinal bacterial flora. The intestinal microbiome is, in fact, nothing more than the set of microbes that live in your intestine (which you may also know by the name "microbiota"), their genetic material, and the interactions they establish with the intestinal environment. And here comes the beauty: maintaining a healthy bacterial flora can help you control your diet and not gain weight.

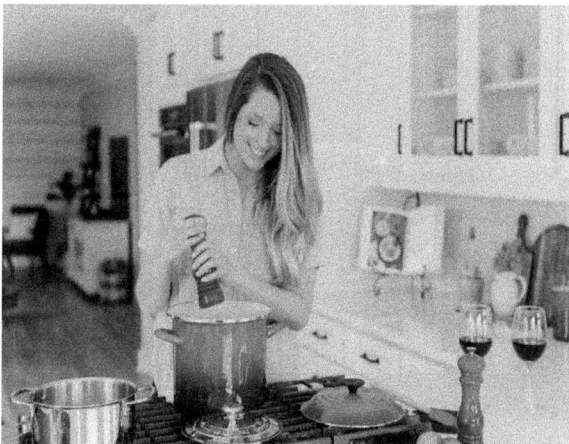

Microbiome diet: how does it work?

I will tell you now to explain how it works the theory supported by the microbiome diet creator, British physician, and science writer Michael Mosley. It is a theory based on numerous scientific evidence that day after day has revealed (and continues to reveal to us) the association between microbiome and health characteristics.

First of all, you need to know that the microbes in your gut participate in your digestion. This means that the amount of energy you can absorb from food also depends on your microbiome.

Second, you also need to know that some bacteria are associated with intestinal inflammation and that intestinal inflammation is associated with obesity. Third, your microbiome communicates with your brain, and that this can lead you to prefer some foods over others. Some studies suggest that by acting on the microbiome's composition, you could reduce your stress levels and sleep better; this could also affect your diet, helping you maintain healthier eating habits.

Foods that are good for the microbiome

The foods that are good for the microbiome are of two types: those containing substances that promote the growth of good bacteria and those that are a source of these bacteria. The former includes foods rich in fiber, such as whole grains, vegetables, fruit, and legumes. The latter are particularly useful because they are rich in soluble fiber, the favorite food of intestinal bacteria. The foods that contain good microbes are fermented foods, such as yogurt, kefir, some cheeses (especially those characterized by a strong smell), fermented vegetables (such as sauerkraut and kimchi), and kombucha (a fermented tea drink).

Other foods, on the other hand, can damage the microbiome. This is the majority of processed foods. Excess sugar, fat, and emulsifiers make them enemies of your intestinal bacteria.

Microbiome diet: an example of a menu

Here is for you an example of a menu for a day of the microbiome diet:

- You can start the day with a yogurt-based breakfast and some fresh fruit.
- At lunch, you can bring legumes to the table, for example, chickpeas in vegetable burgers, accompanied by a mixed salad.
- For dinner, you can make brown rice with vegetables and chicken nuggets.

Remember, though: if you binge, you can't expect to lose weight. The best way to make sure you don't overeat is to have a dietician or nutritionist assess your energy needs.

You must also know that nutrition is not the only component of your lifestyle that can guarantee a healthy microbiome. For this reason, I also advise you to practice adequate physical activity, to avoid smoking, to take antibiotics only when the doctor prescribes them, to try to reduce stress and get enough sleep: these are all useful precautions for the wellbeing of your flora intestinal.

Finally, in case of need, you can rely on probiotic supplements, the bacteria that are allies of health. To be effective, they should provide at least one billion bacteria a day from at least one of the strains contained within them. Again, I invite you to seek advice from an expert before investing any money in buying products.

Under the slogan "diversity matters," the need for the diverse world of microbiomes deserves greater recognition and ceases to be an unknown aspect for citizens is highlighted. To celebrate this day as it deserves, we must understand precisely the microbiome and its relevance in our lives.

Thus, the term microbiome is used to refer to the total number of microorganisms and their genetic material present in humans and is essential for our health.

Gut microbiome and flora

Each human being has a unique microbiome as if it were a fingerprint. Its influence on health and wellbeing is increasingly recognized. According to experts, it has been associated with potential benefits as diverse as improved immune response, reduced risk of obesity or types 2 diabetes, and improved cognition and mood.

If we talk about the human microbiome, we must highlight the flora or intestinal microbiota, the set of bacteria that live throughout our digestive system, especially in the large intestine, and that multiply by millions within us (more than 100 billion bacteria of about 500 to 1,000 different species in a 70 kg adult). Almost all of our microbiota is located in the digestive system.

The diversity of microorganisms, the key to health

Currently, various studies have shown that a greater diversity of microorganisms in our microbiome and, therefore, in the intestinal flora is directly related to health benefits. This is why it is so worrying how, in Western societies, we are suffering a progressive loss of microbial diversity due to busy lifestyles, which can also be associated with an increase in metabolic, immune, and cognitive diseases.

To help maintain the diversity of microorganisms in our body and, consequently, our intestinal flora and our microbiome in normal conditions, we must first attend to our diet. As has been shown, the bacteria that inhabit the intestine depend on the supply of fermentable dietary substrates, which makes the diet a highly relevant factor in the composition of the human intestinal microbiota.

How to have good microbiota?

For this reason, it is important to introduce fiber-rich foods that include prebiotics in our diet. Prebiotics are indigestible compounds, mostly fibers, that serve as food for the bacteria in our digestive system and help us stimulate the microorganisms' growth and activity in our intestinal flora.

A balanced diet is key to getting the recommended daily amount of fiber, including prebiotics. In our day to day, we can find prebiotics in a long list of foods, such as vegetables (artichokes, asparagus, leeks, garlic, onions ...), starches (potatoes and sweet potatoes), fruits (especially bananas), legumes, nuts, and cereals, especially wheat and oats.

It has been shown that increasing the consumption of one of the best-known prebiotics, cereal fiber, helps to achieve good general health and a great diversity in the intestinal microbiota. The intake of between 6-8 g of additional wheat fiber could be enough to generate positive effects on our health.

The microbiome's diet aims to improve the quality of bacteria present in the intestine through food. To understand better, it is first important to know what this microbiome is about. The term refers to the trillions of microorganisms, bacteria, fungi, and viruses that live within our gastrointestinal tract. They act in important functions, such as digestion, the production of hormones, vitamins, other nutrients, and absorption by the body.

And that is how they greatly influence the way the body works and help maintain health. When they are unbalanced, we get sick more often. And that has everything to do with what we eat, since the type and quality of bacteria are defined, among other factors, by our diet.

The exact functioning of the microbiota is still not entirely clear to science. Over the past ten years, researchers have gathered evidence that imbalances between some types of bacteria in the gut favor weight gain. And this is one of the premises of this diet: seeking to achieve balance. Only the task is not simple since no microbiome is the same.

Diet on the shelves

The wave of the microbiome diet started thanks to two books. One was written by Brenda Watson, specializing in gut health and nutrition. Without translation into Portuguese, the work, called *Skinny Gut Diet* (Diet of the Small Intestine) is based on three simple rules:

Eat healthier fats to reduce inflammation

Among these good fats, Watson recommends cold-pressed olive, coconut, and flaxseed oil, in addition to the fat present in food. Like avocados, olives, coconut milk, and salmon. The oils to be avoided are cotton, soy, sunflower, among others, in addition to hydrogenated fat.

Eat live food every day to balance the gut

Among these foods are fermented, starch-free vegetables, and low-sugar fruits. Watson does not prohibit the consumption of dairy products, so yogurts and milk kefir are released.

Eat protein with every meal and snack to avoid binge eating

The proteins indicated by the author are meat, eggs, dairy products, tofu, among others. The second work on the subject was written by the American general practitioner Raphael Kellman and is entitled *The Microbiome Diet* (ed. Cultrix). According to the doctor, a deregulated microbiome can bring a series of problems, such as acne, depression, headache, inflammation, and even fibromyalgia.

The diet proposed in the book has three phases. In the first, which takes 21 days, the goal is to remove unhealthy bacteria from the intestine and replace stomach acids and digestive enzymes. It is the most restricted phase of the entire diet. The adept must cut off all foods, toxins, and chemicals that cause inflammation or imbalance the microbiota. This includes eliminating pesticides, antibiotics, and other drugs. The diet in this phase is based on organic plants and supplements and certain herbs and spices, probiotic and prebiotic foods.

Phase two takes 28 days. Dietary restrictions continue, but less strictly. At this stage, dairy, eggs, vegetables, and gluten-free grains can be taken up. The third phase is considered maintenance and must be followed until the desired weight is lost. According to the doctor, at this stage, the intestine and the microbiota are almost completely balanced. In general, the diet remains the same as in the first and second phases, but in one meal a day, it can eat everything. Almost since processed foods and sugar should still be avoided as much as possible.

Although the microbiome's prominent role in human health has been established, the early-life microbiome is now being recognized as a major influence on human development and long-term health. Variations in the microbiome's composition and functional potential from early life are the result of lifestyle factors such as mode of birth, breastfeeding, diet, and the use of antibiotics. Additionally, variations in the microbiome's composition from early life have been associated with disease-specific outcomes, such as asthma, obesity, and neurodevelopmental disorders. This points towards this bacterial consortium as a mediator between early lifestyle factors and health and disease.

Furthermore, variations in the intrauterine microbial environment can predispose newborns to specific health outcomes later in life. This collective research supports the role of the microbiome in the Developmental Origins of Health and Disease.

Highlighting the critical window of susceptibility in early life associated with the microbiome's development, infant microbial colonization is discussed, beginning with the maternal-fetal exchange of microbes in the uterus and reaching the influence of lactation in the first year of life. Besides, available disease-specific evidence that points to the microbiome as a mediating mechanism in the Developmental Origins of Health and Disease is reviewed.

Sample Microbiome diet list:

Each phase is a little different, but you should add foods that contain probiotics and prebiotics and avoid processed foods in general. Here are some of the foods you should and should eat when you have reached the second phase:

- Vegetables: asparagus; leeks; radishes; the carrots; onion; Garlic; jicama; yams; yam; Sauerkraut, kimchi, and other fermented vegetables
- Fruits: Avocados; rhubarb; apples; the tomatoes; oranges; nectarines; Kiwi; grapefruit; cherries; pears; peaches; mangoes; melons; berries; Coconut
- Dairy products: kefir; Yogurt (or coconut yogurt for a hairless option)
- Grains: Amaranth; buckwheat; Son; gluten-free oats; brown rice Basmati rice; Wild rice
- Fats: nut and seed butter; Beans; Flaxseed, sunflower, and olive oil
- Protein: organic animal protein free from animals in the field; Organic free-range eggs; Fish
- Spices: cinnamon; turmeric

Foods to Avoid in the Microbiome Diet

- Packaged foods
- Gluten
- Soy
- Sugar and artificial sweeteners (Lakanto sweetener is allowed in moderation)
- Trans fats and hydrogenated fats [19659018] Potatoes (except sweet potatoes)
- Corn
- Peanuts
- Meat Deli
- Fish with a high content of mercury

Microbiome Diet Supplements
- Berberine
- Caprylic acid
- Garlic
- Grapefruit seed extract
- Oregano oil
- Wormwood
- Zinc
- Carnosine oil
- Gl9 [Glamamin]

The future of the gut microbiome and nutrition

The human microbiome is incredibly complex and varied. There are many things that we still do not know about the microorganisms that live in the body.

One of the research areas of the microbiota deals with studying the microbiome using "omics" technologies. They are sophisticated techniques that use modern computer systems to analyze large groups of data related to a specific area of biological science.

In the specific case of gut microbiome research, it is interesting to examine the set of genes involved in the microbiome and analyze how the different compounds formed by microorganisms in the gut interact. These technologies help us better understand the amazing variety of microbes that abound in the digestive tract.

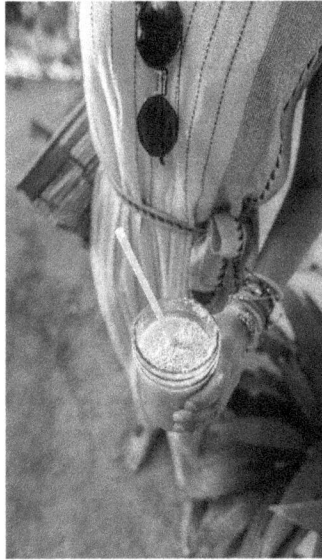

Influence of diet on the intestinal microbiome and its implications for human health

As has already been seen in previous publications, the human intestinal microbiome comprises a set of microorganisms of variable nature and a heterogeneous distribution. Viruses, fungi, and protozoa are an important part of this composition. However, bacteria are the largest and most studied group, predominantly the *Firmicutes* (Gram-positive) and *Bacteroidetes* (Gram-negative) groups.

The numerous beneficial functions that these microorganisms have within the gastrointestinal tract are generally developed in its most distal part, where it accumulates to a great extent and contributes to the synthesis of vitamins, such as K, amino acids, and other products such as the by-products of butyrate, acetate, and propionate, short-chain fatty acids (SCFA), which have an energetic function for epithelial cells, also strengthening the mucosal barrier. On the other hand, the broad relationship between the microbiota and the immune system is known through contact between receptors, metabolites, or the presentation of antigens, inducing a tolerance response or not.

An intestinal environment is a variable place that is highly influenced by different external and internal elements. It has been seen that notable changes in diet or situations of stress and systemic inflammation can generate acute changes in composition pathologies, especially those that cause inflammation at the intestinal level, are associated with a change in the composition, especially of the bacterial fraction, as it is the most studied and predominant, without forgetting that other microorganisms, even when they are to a lesser extent, they can also vary.

It is still difficult to be able to firmly answer whether the disease is the cause or the effect of these changes in the composition, nor is the exact scope of these changes known, but a great relationship between these changes with pathologies such as inflammatory bowel disease, autoimmune diseases such as arthritis, psoriasis and other skin pathologies, showing this strong relationship between the immune system and the microbiome. But, in addition, other pathologies such as obesity, type 2 diabetes, or atherosclerosis also show a drift in bacterial groups.

 In most of these cases, a common consequence of these changes related to SCFA has been detected, decreasing their production, thus reducing their anti-inflammatory, energetic and reinforcing effect on the epithelial cells on the mucosa. In this way, a harmful increase in intestinal permeability could appear, aggravating the consequences. It is also interesting to see how the functionality that the microbiota acquires adapts to the associated pathology. Due to this drift, it suffers as a possible cause or consequence of the disease. It has been seen that in type 2 diabetes, the microbiota of these patients shows an increase in membrane transporters of sugars, branched-chain fatty acids, metabolism of xenobiotic, reduction of sulfate, and decrease in the formation of SCFA and metabolism of cofactors and vitamins. For example, obesity, characterized in a general way with a decrease in the ratio*Bacteroides: Firmicutes*, has shown in studies with mice how this composition increases the ability to extract energy from the diet. Or as when there is an increased risk of atherosclerosis, the microbiota's characterization oscillates towards groups with increased metabolism of proatherogenic components, such as Trimethylamine-N-oxide (TMAO).

The microbiota of a healthy adult tends to be more or less stable over time. Still, all these examples show how, due to a series of circumstances, it can vary in a way that adapts to substantial changes in the environment, which is why many investigations try to understand the true potential of diet in modulating this composition since it is one of the factors involved in the development of the microbiome. Thus, many investigations have focused on studying what differences appear when consuming different macronutrients or, more broadly, different eating patterns, seeing very interesting changes between the bacterial populations present in one or the other situation.

With the development of molecular biology and 16S rRNA sequencing, it has been possible to study in-depth the groups that are present in each circumstance, seeing how protein consumption is related to a general increase in microbial diversity, even depending on the origin, that is, whether it is vegetable or animal, changes in the composition are seen. For this reason, studies using whey protein showed a decrease in *Bacteroides fragilis* and *Clostridium perfringens,* while with pea protein, there was an increase in SCFA production. In both cases, there was an increase in *Bifidobacterium* and *Lactobacillus,* groups of great health interest. In other studies, it was found that animal protein consumption was associated with an increase in *Bacteroides, Biophilia,* and Alistipes, bile-tolerant anaerobes. It would be interesting to deepen these results with more solid research in this regard. There are already results that indicate a great relationship between the type of nutrient and the type of microbiota that develops. It is something logical; each living being has needs. Those who see them covered proliferate, while those who have deficiencies become more vulnerable and tend to disappear or be replaced by others with a greater capacity to adapt to the environment's conditions.

In diets high in protein and low in carbohydrates, a reduction in *Roseburia* and *Eubacterium rectole* has been seen. The detection in feces of a decrease in the production of butyrate and SCFA. In the specific case of red meat, a possible increase in TMAO levels has been seen and, therefore, an increase in the risk of suffering from cardiovascular diseases. Diets high in animal products are usually associated with medium or high-fat intakes, which is why the study of the effects of eating patterns on the composition of the microbiota is much more interesting and real. Regarding the consumption of fats, it has been seen that a diet high in this macronutrient is associated with an increase in the set of anaerobes and *Bacteroides*and, more specifically, if the consumption of saturated fats is high, a relative increase is seen in the proportion of *Faecalibacteriumprausnitzii*, however, when it comes to monounsaturated fats, the drift in the composition is not so remarkable.

But, one of the most studied macronutrients in terms of their relationship with the composition of the microbiota are carbohydrates, which can be degraded by gastrointestinal enzymes to glucose, lactose, or sucrose or, on the other hand, they can be part of non-fibers, digestible and with added benefits.

In diets high in fruits (glucose, fructose, and sucrose), a relative increase of *bifidobacteria* with reduced *Bacteroides* has been seen. But, what is very interesting is what is shown in another study where the addition of lactose is also associated with a decrease in the *Clostridia* group, as well as with lactose supplementation it has measured increases in feces in the concentration of SCFA, for So the elimination of lactose in those tolerant to it may not be entirely beneficial. Of course, it is necessary to expand the research on this to offer clearer conclusions and a much broader perspective.

As for fiber, it is part of the carbohydrates that are not digestible by the gastrointestinal tract enzymes, which is why they reach the intestine practically intact, where the microbiota metabolizes them. Dietary fiber is a source of carbohydrates accessible to the microbiota. In addition to acting many of them as prebiotics, it can also modify the intestinal environment, making it more accessible to beneficial groups for the body.

Among the most relevant prebiotics are soy, inulin, unrefined products, fructans, polydextrose, phosphooligosaccharides (FOS), galactooligosaccharides (GOS), xylooligosaccharides (XOS), and arabinooligosaccharides (OSA), and it has been seen that they promote greater bacterial biodiversity, something very favorable to health, with increases of bifidobacteria and *Lactobacilli*. Specifically, FOS, OSA, and polydextrose are associated with a decrease in *Clostridium* and Enterococcus, and resistant starch promotes *Ruminococcus*, *E. rectole*, and *Roseburia*. On the other hand, the use of probiotics, present in some foods, can also be very interesting, seeing that the addition of fermented dairy products and yogurt can be related to the prevention of inflammatory bowel disease due to certain anti-inflammatory cytokines such as IL-10, in addition to promoting the increase and reduction of more or less beneficial populations, respectively, mentioned above.

As already indicated initially, on a practical level, the interesting thing would be to know how eating patterns modulate the microbiota, beyond specific foods, without neglecting the usefulness of the results offered by studies focused on isolated nutrients, especially to boost the development of new research.

At present, there is a prevalence in our society to acquire nutritional habits with a high amount of animal protein and fat and low fiber content, similar to the so-called Western diet. In these cases, a reduction in both the diversity and beneficial populations of *Bifidobacterium* or *Eubacterium has been seen.* This type of diet is also associated with a greater risk of suffering from other diseases. On the contrary, other diets, such as the Mediterranean, where there is a greater consumption of fruits, vegetables, olive oil, cereals and the intake of animal proteins is moderated, have shown greater diversity as well as greater colonization by beneficial species of *Lactobacillus, Bifidobacterium*, and *Prevotella* with a decrease in *Clostridium.*

It is also remarkable and interesting some results on how also in certain more restrictive diets, such as the gluten-free diet, there are changes in the microbiota's composition towards less beneficial groups, with an increase in *Escherichia coli or Enterobacteriaceae,* as well as other opportunistic pathogens. Although to draw more accurate conclusions, it would be necessary and interesting to know the specific description of the gluten-free diet followed. This fact shows, once again, how the intestinal microbiota is modified according to the environment and the nutrients that arrive.

Whatever the diet is called, and by collecting information on the isolated effects of macronutrients on the microbiota, many investigations show how there is a favorable trend towards developing a healthy intestinal microbiota when ingesting a set of foods, many of the characteristic of a Mediterranean Diet.

And as the saying goes, "all roads lead to Rome," Rome being a healthy diet.

Microbiota and human health

Nutritional based research on the modulation of the intestinal microbiota to improve the state of health and prevent the appearance of certain pathologies, such as obesity, cardiovascular disease or cancer, points to the acquisition of a healthy diet with consumption of fruits, vegetables, whole grains, legumes, and moderate consumption of fish and meat

Not to forget, the adequate intake of polyunsaturated and monounsaturated fats (olive oil).

Every individualized condition will have more specific needs, with dietary adjustments and possible food restrictions for people with intolerances or special requirements, especially in the face of certain pathological states.

In most cases, in general, simply by improving habits towards healthy eating patterns, such as the Mediterranean Diet, there will be improvement in health. This does not mean that we should forget to study intestinal microbiota composition. On the contrary, to know what changes are associated with certain pathologies is quite an important aspect of our daily nutritional regime.

Recent research on the microorganisms changes our understanding of microorganisms as disease-causing agents. Scientists now recognize that the microbiome is an integral part of the human host and integrates with the host's physiology and genetics in a dynamic and bidirectional way—and social on host biology.

We need to consider the impact of social and cultural practices on the microbiome to develop an interconnected and systems approach to approaching public health policy and practice, especially as it applies to the two poles of life: youth and old age.

Recent work carried out by members of the CIFAR Human Microbiome Fellowship emphasizes the importance of using an interdisciplinary research approach to the microbiome's role as part of human wellbeing.

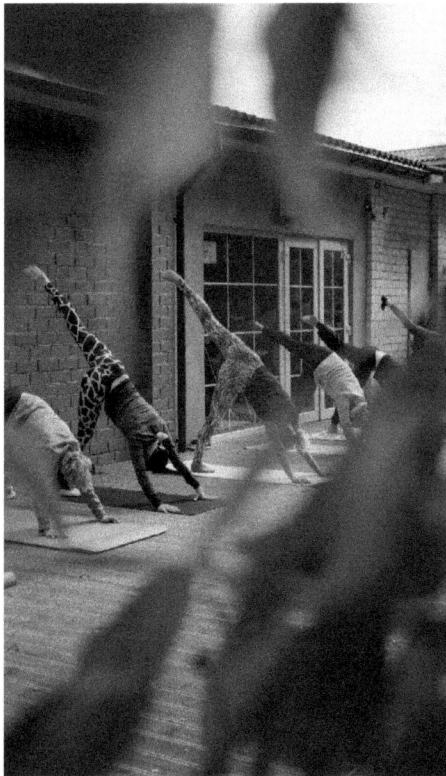

Study results on the human microbiome are relevant for public health experts to recognize when designing services and policies. Studies suggest that social and environmental influences, such as food, exercise, drugs, and climate, can influence the microbiome.

There is a link between improvements in the microbiota and several health effects, like hunger and stunting, because of non-communicable disorders, such as asthma and heart disease, and diseases of age, such as Alzheimer's disease.

A better understanding of the impact of social and environmental influences on health may contribute to additional lines of action for the social determinants of health. Health practitioners must consider the potential impact of clinical practice and health policy on the microbiome.

Greater knowledge of the impact of social and environmental influences on health may contribute to new lines of action concerning the social determinants of health. Clinicians should also consider the potential impact of clinical practice and health policy on the microbiome.

Research by Eran Elinav showed that the microbiota plays a significant role in mediating environmental influences on health outcomes. A genetic correlation was shown to be not the product of the host's genetics but rather a marker in the genetic parentage or genetic markers. Changes in the gut microbiota contribute to variations in the way people respond to allergens by contrast, the genetic variations of the host.

A crucial window is provided for intestinal gut bacteria to modulate host immunity and affect allergies production later in life. Additionally, some bacterial metabolites produced by fiber breakdown tend to defend against allergies. Finally,

The microbiome and communicability of chronic diseases

A team of researchers argues that certain chronic diseases historically thought to be non-communicable, such as non-insulin-dependent diabetes, cardiac disease, and inflammatory bowel disease, may have a transmissible portion via the microbiome, which has significant ramifications for public health concerning prevention measures and care.

The authors address evidence that dysbiosis and pathologies are likely to be caused by a microbiome passed from diseased human or animal models to a non-diseased animal; evidence that when several diseases co-occur within a relatively specific geographic region, they frequently evolve rapidly after implementation of a dysbiotic microbiome; and experimental evidence that the microbiome acquired from a diseased human or animal model may be spread to non-diseased organisms.

Although the association is interesting, it is hard to differentiate the direct influences of environmental influences from the microbiome. They want to spark more discussions and studies to test this more rigorously. The microbiome can affect a chronic disease.

The effect of early antibiotic exposure on wellbeing

An increasing body of research suggests overuse of antibiotics can affect policies and medical practice, particularly the decision to prescribe antibiotics during the newborn age. E-cigarettes raise the risk of contracting asthma.

Brett Finlay and colleagues provided evidence from the prospective cohort study Canadian Stable Baby Longitudinal Development (CHILD) Study affecting approximately 3,500 children followed since before birth. Low diversity in the gut microbiome and a high risk of asthma are seen in children who received systemic antibiotics during the first year of life.

A new study from Martin Blaser's lab offers more proof that early antibiotic use impacts health effects later in life. Baby mice exposed to antibiotics from their mother's milk experienced more serious colitis when infected with a pathogenic strain of an intestinal bacteria 80 days after the exposure. In these mice, the microbiota was distinct and applied to an axenic mouse that was not exposed to antibiotics in their early life, resulted in a similar susceptibility to a more severe type of colitis.

Connecting growth with the microbiome

In a study, researchers studied children's microbiota against the backdrop of stunted growth, a significant public health issue affecting a quarter of the world's children. By studying the fecal and gut microbiomes of more than 400 children in Madagascar and the Central African Republic, the analysis showed that the bacteria in the upper gut mimic the stomach's bacteria. It is typically contained in the mouth and esophagus.

It also decreased the number of types of bacteria that manufacture butyrate, a nutrient-rich metabolite, and increased the types of bacteria that cause enteroathogenic infections. This research finds that a protein causes growth retardation in brain cells.

Gut bacteria and probiotics

Probiotics are widely common as a food supplement or as a medication. The true health advantages of probiotics and their side effects are also mostly poorly known. A research was published by Eran Elinav and colleagues that explores how probiotics affect the regeneration of the gut microbiome after antibiotic therapy.

Volunteers obtained a broad-spectrum antibiotic treatment and were given either an autologous fecal transplant (fecal sample taken from them before antibiotics and passed back to their gut) or were allowed to heal spontaneously. The recipients who had undergone an autologous fecal transplant within a day recovered initial 'native' microbiota, while those who recovered by themselves took three weeks.

However, no matter how many probiotics were successfully inserted in the intestine, the microbiota did not return to its natural state for at least five months. This research shows there is a substantial tradeoff to remember when using probiotics after antibiotic therapy.

Autologous fecal transplantation presents logistic challenges, but further research may reveal the particular components of an individual microbiome that contribute to the development of personalized probiotic treatment.

This research indicates there is a substantial tradeoff to consider when using probiotics after antibiotic therapy. Research can recognize particular components of individual microbiomes that may lead to creating a well-circumscribed and personalized probiotic treatment.

The role of the microbiome in age-related diseases

A review article published in Bioessays by Brett Finlay, Sven Pettersson, Melissa Melby, and Thomas Bosch summarizes the many connections between the microbiome and aging, which may have significant consequences aging population, and their effect on the healthcare system.

Studies show that the growth factor FGF21 – responsible for regulating host metabolism and longevity - is regulated by the gut microbiome, and animal experiments suggest transplanting young microbiomes into old mice may enhance longevity.

Metabolites formed by these types of processes may be affected by lifestyle factors. Many other factors affect psychological and behavioral responses to aging by their effects on the gut and brain chemicals production.

One example is that a diet high in soy increases longevity and a more favorable experience of menopause among the Japanese.

In another recent research, the suggestion that the microbiome plays a role in developing Alzheimer's disease was confirmed. Mice genetically bred to be more resistant to Alzheimer's symptoms appear to have lower microbe levels that make essential vitamins. If mice are placed on a calorie-restricted diet, these microbes start to come back.

Compared to their normal counterparts, mice on a calorie-restricted diet had fewer amyloid β plaques in the brain. Also, they had a lower expression of pro-inflammatory genes in the gut. When mice were fed such bacterial strains that were the most likely to cause an increase in the brain, they found that there was an increase in amyloid plaques in the brain, possibly through the gut-brain axis.

 If findings are repeated in humans, diet can be a mode of action against Alzheimer's disease. It is important to note that female mice did not exhibit these results. They found that plaques grew in size, indicating a direct biological impact that could be occurring along the gut-brain axis. If findings are repeated in humans, diet can be a mode of action against Alzheimer's disease.

It is important to remember that there were no significant effects on males. They found that amyloid β plaques' size increased, indicating a direct biological effect occurring through the gut-brain axis. If findings are repeated in humans, diet can be a mode of action against Alzheimer's disease. These results were only seen in female mice, but not in males.

Next steps

The Human Microbiome Program has established key questions or research directions that may further explain the microbiome's function in human health and the degree to which it acts as a mediator or buffers for the effects of environmental factors.

- Better determination of the causal role of microorganisms in health and disease.
- The researchers hope to establish genetic factors that help microbiota health.
- There is a continued study of the microbiome in other areas beyond the intestine.
- Ongoing studies will continue to investigate the microbiota and its relationship to the E. coli findings.

Improving your gut flora

The gut is the pillar of good health and general wellbeing. It is essential because it is an organ that needs its ecosystem. Our intestinal flora produces 80% of our immune cells, which help to protect us from diseases.

Keep in mind that our digestive tract represents our overall health, so it's important to take care of it to be the best version of yourself. Strong gut health and overall wellbeing are two sides of the same coin. A balanced gut biome is vital to the immune system. The best support for bacteria is a daily diet that includes probiotics and prebiotics.

The discrepancy between probiotic and prebiotic

"Probiotic" is also used to refer to "prebiotic" I want you to get a little acquainted with it. Prebiotics are soluble foods of plant origin that the human body is not able to digest. They are vital for promoting the growth of beneficial bacteria in the gut. Legumes (i.e., beans) are the food we can explore later.

Probiotics, also known as "good bacteria," are live microorganisms that bind themselves to the intestinal flora. You must ensure a safe and balanced digestive system by consuming both prebiotics and probiotics. It helps with bowel movements and relieves constipation and diarrhea. A solution to all of this occurs with traditional food products.

The digestive tract is divided into many parts. The intestinal system is the most critical component of our immune system. The large intestine is responsible for immune response, but it also maintains the body's water and mineral balance. The small intestine is where much of the digestion occurs and is the organ responsible for absorbing nutrients. A patient may have filtering nutrients continuously.

Intestines assist in consuming nutrients and at the same time keep bacteria, fungi, and other pathogens at bay. In addition to doing continuous surveillance work, the healthy gut can also recognize toxins and flush them out of the body.

The human microbiome is a genus of good bacteria that we can have in our diet and supplement. The microbiome is a collection of all the microorganisms that live inside and outside the skin. It is estimated that there are around 100 billion bacteria in total.

The human microbiome consists of several microorganisms. These involve many bacteria, viruses, and fungi. The gut microbiome is essential to our digestive organs. It is important to make sure that the food we consume is cooked properly, which also helps our gut and body.

The microbiome synthesizes vitamins B1, B2, B12, and vitamin K, which are short-chain fatty acids that serve as an energy source for the intestinal mucosa cells and promote intestinal mobility. The gut microbiota assists in immune response, detoxification, and control of inflammation.

Then, this little helper aids our immune system to combat diseases and also contributes to our body.

How can I help my intestinal flora survive?

A balanced diet encourages a healthy intestinal microbiome. Fermented vegetables are particularly easy to prepare and provide a good basis for a diet. Those with compromised gut flora should start here.

What should I do to better my health?

One thing that can help boost gut health is exercise. Get enough sleep. And most importantly, eat a balanced diet. Gut friendly diet is the most important factor and is easy to achieve. We will also explore a balanced diet below. There is another rule: It is important to eat a well-balanced diet, avoid stress, and stop taking some medications.

Try to keep the intestinal flora up

There are some positive improvements you can bring to your gut wellbeing. Having enough sleep will make you feel more refreshed and be in good physical shape. When you are still tired, your body cannot relax properly. This makes it more likely the illness will gain an advantage over you. It is recommended that you rub your stomach regularly to help it pass through. It acts to calm the gut in a targeted way and reduces tension.

Regular physical activity should be part of your everyday life because exercise is an essential factor in improving your intestinal flora. Some drugs have been found to interact with the intestinal flora.

They produce inflammation and, because they affect both "good" intestinal bacteria and the one to be eradicated, they can cause diarrhea. Stop alcohol and tobacco use, minimize tension, and consider other causes so that you avoid the risk of developing disorders such as irritable bowel syndrome 3.

A healthy diet is important for maintaining good intestinal health. For this project, we will be looking into beneficial foods that are particularly beneficial to the gut. It is really necessary to consume nutritious foods. The value of a diet that enhances gut health is not limited to the gut. Read on to try new dishes.

What foods support the intestine?

Some foods are ideal for intestinal health. It is important to increase the consumption of probiotics and prebiotics in our diet. Both are important to improve the intestinal ecosystem.

Fermented foods are advantageous. However, as long as you consume the food peacefully, it does not impose stress on your body—slow and leisurely chewing.

What is fermentation?

What happens when we ferment food? Fermented foods go through a transition in their metabolism as they are cultured by fungi and cells (microorganisms). Fermentation is the operation. Fermented foods should be consumed immediately after preparation since beneficial bacteria die after a certain amount of time. Fermented foods are gut-friendly foods and can be enjoyed in several ways. There are several choices when selecting fermented foods.

Foods to avoid to improve gut wellbeing

The food/chemical you select may affect the intestinal flora. It lets you choose the right foods for your stomach. Gluten and fast-absorbing carbohydrates should be avoided as much as possible. Gluten is also hard to digest because the protein structure is very compact. Sugar encourages the growth of fungi and yeasts and the proliferation of harmful intestinal bacteria. In certain cases, it contributes to inflammation. Processed or fried fats, including sausages and smoked meats, are not good for the stomach. Some packaged and ultra-processed foods should be avoided because of their additives. It is important to know that a healthy body can withstand a moderate intake of coffee and alcohol. It may cause a laxative effect and cause diarrhea if ingested in excess. Coffee and alcohol can cause gas (flatulence), which is bad for your stomach.

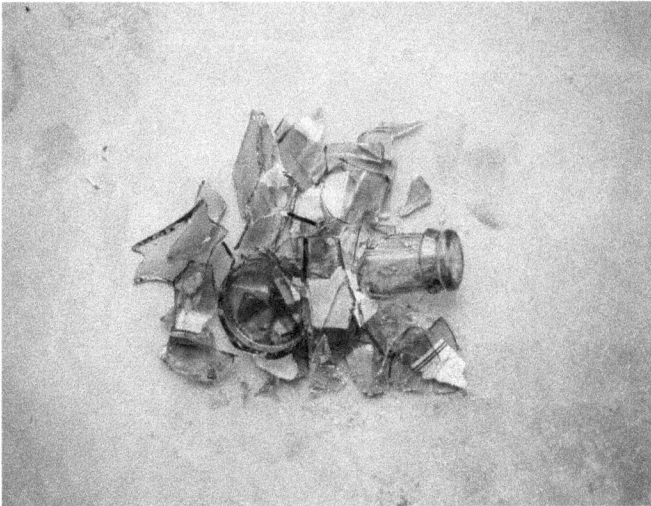

Cooking for a balanced gut

With the previous tips on a safe diet for the intestine, we can give you some healthy cooking strategies at home to practice to adopt a balanced diet.

- Eat meat just twice a week. Try the flexitarian diet.
- Use raw meats and particularly offal products such as sausage.

- Reduce your grain consumption. Wheat, barley, and oats produce a lot of gluten.
- If you have the chance, purchase fresh eggs, meat, and other products from direct suppliers. They are likely more wholesome than industrially manufactured products.
- Using coconut, olive, or rapeseed oil for cooking. Use butter instead of margarine.
- Eat foods that are normal and don't visit the ultra-processed foods.
- Eat dairy products in moderation. You will have to judge by your tolerance level what is the appropriate number.
- In this context, there are no drawbacks to cooking dishes that contain vegetables.
- Include whole-grain foods in your diet. Taking this will help you get a lot of dietary fiber.

If your stomach is sensitive, pay attention to what you eat in general. If you eat items of animal origin, you should particularly consider the highest quality. Shop from a direct source and help local trade, which is not commercial. Be conscious of foods that you can avoid if you have food allergies or intolerances. It can be frustrating when it comes to safe dietary choices. We know that it is often difficult to find the best way to lead your life, but by paying attention to your health and following our advice, you will always find the right direction.

Nourishing the intestine by physical activity

Also mentioned above, physical activity plays an important role in the healthy intestinal flora. Exercise is the perfect way to keep the digestive system in tip-top condition. Certain sports can maintain a balanced stomach, like cycling, swimming, and track and field.

Again, get enough exercise. It avoids constipation and bloating and helps your intestine function better. A balanced gut will make for better athletic results.

Researchers have discovered a correlation between certain diseases and the changes that the gut microbiome undergoes. These diseases also include inflammatory bowel diseases, obesity, diabetes mellitus, some types of autism, Alzheimer's, and variant sclerosis.

For these reasons, living a balanced lifestyle and consuming a nutritious diet should be emphasized. You now have all the vital knowledge you need to adopt a safe lifestyle.

Take control of your gut for your good.Proper intestinal health requires daily maintenance.

You will benefit from a diet rich in prebiotics and probiotics, and your immune system will function more effectively. Do not push yourself to accomplish this aim. Receive help and encourage yourself to indulge once in a while. A safe lifestyle doesn't automatically involve giving up all.

A balanced balance between personal satisfaction and a healthy digestive system will establish a rewarding and healthy life. Your mood will affect your gut health and diet. You will learn more about this by looking at the word "nutritional psychiatry."

Is the western diet permanently damaging our health?

It was thought that what happens inside our gut could affect our overall health. Researchers have found that the gut microbiome influences whether the brain will be stimulated by nicotine.

Your gut's microbiota is made up of thousands of microbes. These tiny organisms are present at birth and are shaped by genetics and other factors throughout life.

The digestive tract can be likened to a small garden. Microbes on the skin interact with the human body and have implications for energy harvesting, immune system education, and chronic inflammatory diseases. Dr. Sam Smits of Stanford University told Healthline, an online publication.

It's healthy to eat a healthy diet.

In the last century, the human diet has changed drastically. Changes in diet, especially the introduction of antibiotics, cesarean deliveries, increased sedentary activity, and the replacement of fruits and vegetables with fiber-free processed options, have led to a major shift in human health.

To see how diet impacts our microbiome, researchers studied a hunter-gatherers group in Tanzania known as the Hadza.

"In the modern industrialized world, we have the opportunity to learn about the shapes of our remote human ancestors," said Justin Sonnenburg, Ph.D., associate professor of microbiology and immunology.

The Hadza hunter-gatherer group has a diet consisting of meat, berries, tubers, and honey. Their diet is more at the mercy of the seasons in the dry season, and berries are a more important part of their diet in the wet season.

The researchers found that gut microbiota in the Hadza is different and more diverse than industrialized humans. Besides, the specific types of bacteria present in the Hadza in the dry season have become almost completely extinct in most people living in the industrialized world.

According to Dr. Eugene Chang, AGAF, a member of the American Gastroenterological Association Center for Gut Microbiome Research and Education, it matters if those in the Western world miss some of these microbial species. Those who eat a Western diet may be losing key microbial species that are important for maintaining health. And these microbes are lost because of the diet. Therefore, key microbes are lost, and imbalances and the absence of key microbes are observed.

Recently there has been a lot of research suggesting that gut health plays an important role in overall wellbeing. There is evidence that the composition of the microbiota is different between the traditional and industrialized populations. There is evidence for an increase in chronic diseases in Western populations. We know that the microbiome is involved in many of these diseases. Together, these studies suggest that the microbiota in industrialized populations do not protect against these diseases.

Gut health is linked to many diseases: If the gut microbiome becomes abnormal, it can have significant effects on overall health. These chemicals can negatively affect your immune system and metabolism, leading to inflammatory bowel disease, type 1 diabetes, liver disease, obesity, malnutrition, and diabetes.

A 2016 study also led by Sonnenburg showed that dietary fiber greatly reduces the diversity of gut microbes. There was increased fiber in the diet. If fiber deprivation was maintained for four generations, the microbial species that recovered were permanently lost.

The evolution of our diet might be similar to what is happening in the guts of those in the Western world. Hunter-gatherers lived on what was available. Diet was limited to what was available at the time, leading to variation in gut microbes. We are less reliant on finding food in modern western societies. We can go to the grocery store, pick up various products, and buy them whenever we want. Our choices are often guided by convenient, economical, prepared, packaged, processed, high-fat, high-calorie, low-fiber, and low-cost foods.

Many people who eat a traditional African diet are healthier than people in the Western world because they eat lots of vegetables and fiber. The Hadza get a lot of fiber in their diet. We consume around 15 grams per day. However, making sure our gut microbes get back to our old ways may not be as easy as emulating the Hadza diet. Changing the diets and lifestyles of people in Western countries is not possible because they won't. "However, we may be able to replenish the missing components in your gut microbiome and keep them on hand by supplementing their diets with certain types and sufficient amounts of dietary fiber supplements, using microbiome analysis to determine how this regimen can be adjusted."

Chapter 6: Mediterranean Diet—the game changer

It is the new year, and we are all full of resolutions, many of them related to dieting, so we offer you this excellent, nutritious, and delicious option...

The Mediterranean Diet corresponds to the eating pattern of the island of Crete, part of Greece and southern Italy, at the beginning of the sixties, that is where it originated; This type of diet is considered a reference for a healthy diet and is recommended in various countries due to the health benefits it provides.

The diet in the Mediterranean regions is identified by the following common components, also known as the decalogue of the Mediterranean diet:

1. Use olive oil as the main additional fat: it is traditionally used for preparing and dressing meals.

2. Eat plenty of plant-based foods: fruits, vegetables, legumes, mushrooms, and nuts: Vegetables should be present at lunch and dinner, approximately two servings at each meal. At least one of them must be raw.

3. Bread and foods from cereals (pasta, rice, and especially their whole-grain products) should be part of the daily diet: One or two servings per meal should preferably be whole since some nutrients (magnesium, phosphorus, etc.) and fiber can be lost in processing.

4. The little processed, fresh, and seasonal foods are the most suitable; Without a doubt, the more natural foods are, the more benefits they will bring us.

5. Consume dairy products moderately daily, mainly yogurt and cheeses, due to prebiotics' high content to strengthen the intestinal flora.

6. Red meat should be consumed in moderation and if it can be as part of stews and other recipes—processed meats in very small quantities and as ingredients in snacks and dishes.

7. Eat plenty of fish and eggs in moderation.

8. Fresh fruit should be the usual dessert. Sweets and cakes should be eaten occasionally, as traditional desserts contain worrying amounts of refined sugar and flour.

9. Water is the drink par excellence in the Mediterranean. The usual consumption is 1.5 to 3 liters a day, depending on weight, height, and physical activity level. Wine should be taken in moderation and during meals is good for digestion.

10. Do physical activity every day, as it is just as important as eating properly.

As we have already been saying, this type of diet stands out, particularly for the nutritional benefits it offers. These are some examples:

Olive oil is rich in vitamin E, beta-carotene, and monounsaturated fatty acids, which is why it has cardio protective properties (it protects our heart).

Due to the high consumption of fruits and vegetables and its high content of antioxidants and fiber, this diet helps prevent some cardiovascular diseases and some types of cancer, especially breast, ovarian, esophagus, and stomach.

Oleic acid is considered an antithrombotic agent (prevents clots in arteries or veins), unlike saturated fatty acids.

Folic acid, contained in some kinds of vegetables, can reduce homocysteine levels, identified as one of the risk factors in cardiovascular disease.

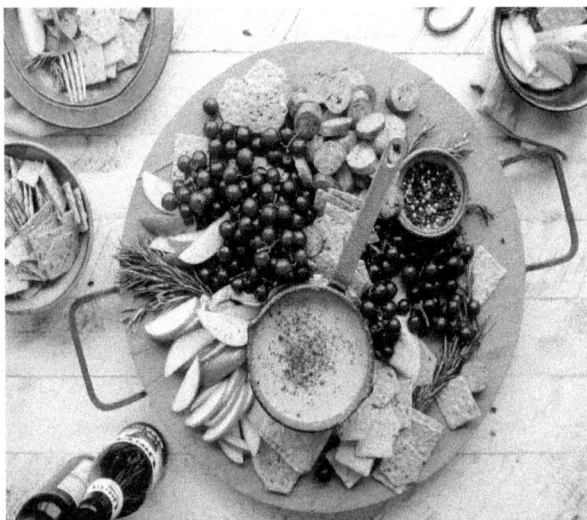

Reducing the amount of salt in the diet reduces blood pressure; it is recommended to keep your salt intake below 5 g per day, equivalent to one teaspoon. The foods with the highest amount of salt are bouillon cubes, commercial soups, salted cod, cured pork bacon, pizzas, precooked (croquettes, dumplings), blue cheese, ketchup, serrano ham, olives and pickles, cooked ham, cheese Manchego, commercial French fries, salty nuts, and all kinds of sausages.

Plant protein helps the biosynthesis of vitamins and amino acids, the breakdown of sugar alcohols, and ammonia's excretion. In contrast, protein derived from animals and plants acts oppositely in the intestinal microbiota.

Fortunately, we have the ability and opportunity to choose the foods we want to consume, from a wide variety; It is our responsibility to choose wisely, making small changes in our eating habits, which will be reflected in our health. It is in this way that we are solely responsible for our state of health. Let's avoid blaming our family, friends, society, doctors, government, hospitals, or finances; we choose what we eat. Our habits are reflected in our quality of life.

If it is difficult for you to make changes, remember that experts in the nutritional and nutritional areas can advise. Turn to an experienced nutritionist so they can clarify your doubts and guide you regarding your food intake. We can support you since it is a complimentary area for the health of all our patients and their families.

And as Hippocrates said in the past:

"May thy food be thy medicine, and may thy medicine be thy food."

Listen to your Grandma

How many times have you heard your grandmother say that the Mediterranean diet is the best? But do you know what it means? And do you know?

One of the main debates in the world of nutrition is the one that encompasses the Mediterranean diet, and the truth is that there is no clear definition of the concept, so it lends itself to multiple interpretations. The latter can lead to misuse of the term at the textual level and the food level.

Let's go with a little history

Before starting to discuss the risks or benefits of the famous "Mediterranean diet," as well as providing the term with a definition as objective as possible, it is interesting to place the concept in history, discover its origin, because to a certain extent, *we are what in each moment we live.* The nutritionist and biologist Juan Revenga, professor at the University of San Jorge in Zaragoza and author of the blog "El Nutrionista de la General," reveals the concept's origin through the Study *of the Seven Countries.*

To carry out the latter, the American physiologist Ancel Keys took as a sample 7 countries of the Mediterranean basin (Italy, Greece, former Yugoslavia, the Netherlands, Finland, Japan, and the USA) and carried out a continuous study of the different lifestyles including diet as a key factor. He discovered that these countries had better health, and it was all because of one factor: diet.

As a result of the analysis results carried out in the middle of the 20th century, the concept of "Mediterranean diet" was born.

Does it have a place in the 21st century?

Quoting Juan Revenga, "the Mediterranean diet is not chosen, it is chosen, it depends on the circumstances. It is not chosen. It is associated with a historical moment. We can choose specific nuances". To understand it, we could parallel with the political transition: that moment in the history of a country in which it goes from authoritarian regimes to established democracies, since the same happens in the nutritional transition.

But then, could we currently carry out a Mediterranean diet? Yes, but we would have to say goodbye to many things that we will not give up now. We can make a kind of "*Mediterranean makeup,* "that is, always include seasonal things, do the shopping in the market, cook more.

Benefits

According to the European Food Safety Authority (EFSA), and as Juan Revenga explained to us, "it cannot be said that the Mediterranean diet is a concept to which health benefits can be transferred for two reasons: it is not an element that is fully defined, everyone can interpret it in their way. And "includes wine," which is an alcoholic beverage.

However, if we ignore these elements and focus mainly on the pattern where the dominance of abundant consumption of fruits, vegetables, and vegetables can be appreciated, it would be beneficial. And, as Aitor Sánchez argues, of what is known and there is more scientific abundance, and "for what the Mediterranean diet is most recommended is to prevent cardiovascular risk or other non-communicable diseases also associated with cardiovascular risk (hypertension, diabetes types 2) or to prevent different types of cancer and of course also for neurodegenerative diseases because of the protector that healthy fats can present ". Of all this is what today is most studied the Mediterranean dietary pattern.

All the world's culinary traditions have something to offer, whether they delight the palate or enhance our health. Or both at the same time, as happens with the Mediterranean diet: that which, according to many nutritional experts, is the best diet in the world. But why? Is it the ingredients? The combinations? Or, is it not rather the way of eating of Europeans?

That does not mean that we should renounce one of the —few— whims of globalization, which is to be able to try dishes and ingredients from almost any region of the world, much less that we renounce the diet of our own country, which like all of them, it is a treasure and part of our identity. Rather, checking why the Mediterranean diet is the best can help us convince ourselves to add its benefits to our diet, making the most of it - something that is good to do with all the world's diets.

Various studies give for the Mediterranean diet to be the best because it works as preventive medicine for a range of conditions. It is also capable of taking better care of two of our most important organs than other diets: the heart and the brain. This promotes a better and longer life.

The secret of the Mediterranean diet

The first thing that stands out about this diet, full of vegetables, cereals, bread, seeds, and fats from various sources, such as fish and olive oil, is that it is not exactly "light." According to a study conducted by the US National Institute of Public Health, the inhabitants of Mediterranean countries consume more fat than Americans. However, this intake comes from monounsaturated and polyunsaturated fats, present in eating habits that promote a long and healthy life.

This is one of the things that make the Mediterranean diet the best, and more so in these times when much of the processed food is full of saturated fats that, in excess, produce cardiovascular and even cognitive problems. This has caused many to fear any type of fat and completely omit it from their diet. However, what you have to do is include good fats, such as those present in the Mediterranean diet.

Benefits for the heart and brain

According to dietitian Victoria Taylor, from the British Heart Foundation, for the BBC, a large amount of research on the Mediterranean diet has shown that it prevents all kinds of conditions: from type 2 diabetes to high blood pressure and high cholesterol. All of these are risk factors for the heart, so without a doubt, a Mediterranean diet helps to evolve this vital organ.

As research on the benefits of this type of diet progresses, it may be increasingly revealed that certain foods are of greater importance to health. For now, however, it appears that it is the general diet and food combining approach, rather than the "superfoods" alone, that makes this a healthy way to eat.

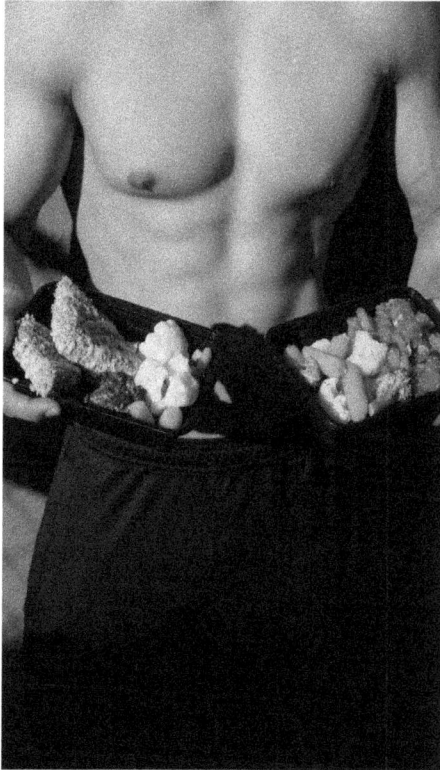

However, this specialist highlights that it is good to add elements of the Mediterranean diet to our eating habits. Just making the transition from saturated fats to mono and polyunsaturated fats is already quite beneficial, even if our diet is not completely Mediterranean. So adding fish, nuts, and olive oil to your dishes is something you can try little by little to strengthen your heart… and also your brain.

As confirmed by a group of researchers from the National Autonomous University of Mexico, although saturated fats are addictive and can interfere with the prefrontal cortex's functioning, the good fats present in the foods help prevent the deterioration of cognitive functions. They may even reduce the risk of Alzheimer's.

In recent years, epidemiological and clinical studies have provided a solid scientific basis on the beneficial effects of the Mediterranean diet in preventing cardiovascular diseases and other chronic diet-related diseases, including some types of cancer.

Numerous scientific studies have pointed out the reasons why olive oil is preferable from a health point of view to other types of fat and even other types of vegetable oils:

Oleic acid is considered an antithrombotic agent compared to saturated fatty acids.

Most intervention studies on cardiovascular disease have shown that saturated acids are atherogenic, while monounsaturated fatty acids lower total cholesterol levels. But just as monounsaturated fatty acids (and also olive oil) produce a decrease in LDL-cholesterol levels (a risk factor in cardiovascular diseases) and maintain plasma HDL-cholesterol levels (protective factor), acids Polyunsaturated fats only lower LDL-cholesterol.

Concerning polyunsaturated fatty acids, oleic acid has the advantage that it is more resistant to oxidative phenomena, which is beneficial given the involvement of oxidative processes in atherosclerosis development.

Olive oil provides antioxidants such as vitamin E and phenolic compounds.

Likewise, the abundance of plant origin foods in the Mediterranean diet ensures a sufficient supply of a wide variety of essential micronutrients (vitamins and minerals), fiber, and other substances present in vegetables with known beneficial effects on health. For example, folic acid in some kinds of vegetables can reduce homocysteine levels, which is identified as one of the risk factors in cardiovascular disease.

Moderate alcohol consumption is also known to lower cardiovascular disease risk, probably by increasing HDL-cholesterol levels. However, it should not be forgotten that the recommendations on the beneficial effects of wine must always be accompanied by a warning about the dangers of alcohol abuse on health.

Finally, the contribution of antioxidants in both fruits and vegetables and olive oil (rich in vitamin E) or red wine reduces the risk of cardiovascular disease.

The high consumption of fruits and vegetables in the Mediterranean diet may reduce the risk of certain types of cancer, especially of the esophagus and stomach. Recent studies have also pointed to a possible preventive role of olive oil in certain types of cancer such as breast and ovarian cancer.

Nutritional pyramid

In 1993, scientists gathered at the International Conference on Mediterranean Diets to review the scientific research carried out so far on the composition of the Mediterranean diet and its effects on health, developed a nutritional pyramid to reflect the characteristic dietary habits of the Mediterranean. Mediterranean diet as a reference diet.

This pyramid's objective was to graphically represent the relative proportions, the frequency, and the approximate servings of the food groups that contribute to the food model that constitutes the

Mediterranean diet. This pyramid is a dietary guide for the healthy adult population and should be modified for special population groups such as children and pregnant women.

It reflects the recommendation on moderate alcohol consumption, defined as the intake of 1 to 2 glasses of wine per day for men and one glass per day for women.

Life philosophy

In short, the Mediterranean diet as a reference diet has a beneficial effect on health. It is difficult to determine the beneficial effect of olive oil rich in oleic acid and vitamin E or that attributable to other foods such as fish, cereals, or legumes within the Mediterranean diet.

Therefore, one should think about the Mediterranean diet as a whole, in which the beneficial effects of the different components are surely additive or synergistic. Since the substances with beneficial effects are present in different foods in variable amounts, today, almost all dietary guidelines emphasize the importance of consuming a highly varied diet that incorporates a large number of unprocessed foods such as fresh fruits and vegetables.

Likewise, when judging the positive effects of the Mediterranean diet, we must not forget the role that other non-dietary factors related to the Mediterranean regions' culture possibly play in the low incidence of chronic diseases, such as a calmer life, less stress, nap, etc.

The authentic Mediterranean Diet has 15 foods—get to know all!

The Mediterranean Diet is abundant in herbs, fruits, and nuts. Do you know which ones? We will discover 15 local foods or have been part of our society for centuries.

Wheat

Cereal (grow) is the essential pillar of the Mediterranean diet. Even though wheat is not king, bread is king. If you don't have a gluten allergy, it is a safe meal. It is a great source of essential nutrients that give you energy and keep you safe. These products can be used in some types such as bread, flour, pasta, batters (the latter is considered a superfood because of the nutrients it contains).

Olive oil

Olive oil is an emblematic food of the Mediterranean Diet. Olive tree cultivation is one of the oldest in this region, dating back 4,000 years before Christ. He is a good guy. Numerous studies indicate it can prevent breast cancer or reduce cholesterol (reduces bad cholesterol and increases good). The essential oil is important because it is more expensive. If refined, it loses its protective virtues.

Use it both for cooking and dressing. However, it is caloric: one tablespoon (10 ml) contains 90 kcal.

Garlic and onion

Greeks and Romans claimed that onions and garlic had medicinal powers and have been eaten in many of the dishes from the Mediterranean diet.

The purple onion variety has the most quercetin, a material with anti-inflammatory and analgesic activity.

Garlic, besides improving the flavor of any stew, is one of the strongest natural antibiotics. Regular intake of more than 10g of garlic has been shown to lower the risk of cancer.

Peppers

This food item has now become an important part of our dietary habits. It is an obligatory ingredient in stir-fries and recipes such as the escalivada (pepper, eggplant, and onion in the oven). Red peppers contain triple the amount of vitamin C of oranges.

The supplement also includes massive doses of the antioxidant zeaxanthin.

Lettuce

It is the star of all Mediterranean salads. Caesar Salad's roots may date back to the time of the Romans, who served lettuce at all meals. Vitamin A should be eaten regularly since it has a long list of nutrients. And no energy costs.Chew it well though.

Carrot

Wild carrots have been grown in the Mediterranean for a long time. This is why they are an important part of the Mediterranean Diet. Beta-carotene or Vitamin A is the richest vegetable in the vitamin A family. It is a natural anti-diarrheal that calms stomach pain and fights diarrhea.

Tomatoes

Tomato soup has been a common part of many cultures. It is an essential factor in stir-fries and salads. The fruit is a great source of lycopene, an antioxidant that fights free radicals, protecting against diseases, including cancer.

Using virgin olive oil with tomato sauce to make your tomato sauce even more nutritious.

Legumes

In the Mediterranean region, lentils and peas are eaten in ancient times. Legumes were appreciated by both the Greeks and the Romans. Beans come from America but are also heavily incorporated into our diet. Legumes contain nutrition as well as the essential amino acids that the body requires. They are excellent sources of slow-absorbing carbohydrates and fiber.

Fish

Fish is another of the diet's compulsory foods. A large variety of fish is recommended, but we would choose the sardine.

It is popular and inexpensive. Although it is a "second-rate fish," it has high omega-three fats, which is why it is an ally of cardiovascular health.

Seafood is more common in Mediterranean diets. The most consumed meat was poultry (white meat). The diet contained red meat due to the influence of Germanic peoples, but it was not a traditional Mediterranean diet.

White meat has less saturated fat and cholesterol than red meat. Birds are also good choices.

Figs

Olive trees and fig trees are a great part of the Mediterranean's essence. The consumption of wine has existed in this region since time immemorial.

Resveratrol is an effective antioxidant that battles the destructive action of free radicals and protects your cells.

And dried figs contain a lot of calcium: 35 mg/100 g of dried food if fresh and 162 mg/100 g of dry food if dried.

Cabbage family

Examples of vegetables in the Mediterranean Diet are broccoli, cauliflower, and turnips. Ideal for steaming, boiling, or producing broth.

Crucifers contain compounds like Indole-3-carbinol (found in cauliflower) and sulforaphane (found in broccoli).

The positive thing about steam is that it detoxifies your body.

Oranges

It first came from the East in the 10th century and has ended up being one of the most common fruits in the Mediterranean region. Taking vitamin C in juice is a tasty way to acquire vitamin C. A nutrient to shield you from infection. Additionally, it is advisable in people with anemia since it is best absorbed. Oranges also flush uric acid from the body.

Almonds and hazelnuts

The hazelnut has been grown in the Mediterranean region for decades. Spain is a major producer of hazelnuts. They also have regional requirements. They are high in oleic acid and vitamin E (a powerful antioxidant).

Almonds were grown in Persia, then introduced to Spain. In the Medieval period, they were eaten in Spain, and then they were grown in the Mediterranean. It contains a lot of calcium and vitamin D, so it is an alternative to milk.

Greek yogurt

While the most common Greek yogurt is produced in Greece, the dairy originates in Turkey. Yogurt is easier to digest, has less fat, and contains healthy bacteria that balance the gut microbiome. The balance of a balanced microbiota is important for good general health.

A lot of scientific research highlights the advantages of the Mediterranean Diet. It has been shown to help fend off cancer and maintain cardiovascular health. But what is the secret to its many benefits?

The advantages of the Mediterranean Diet are found in these components: this form of diet consists of olive oil, fatty fish, and nuts.

The proportions of their dishes are cereal and vegetables as the basis, and meats or similar only as a garnish. Micro-nutrients are present due to the use of seasonal vegetables, aromatic herbs, and seasonings.

UNESCO has recognized the Mediterranean Diet as an intangible cultural heritage of humanity.

Get some nutritional discipline

Eating and nourishing are two different things, although closely related. **We need** knowledge about food and mental, emotional, and corporal **discipline** to nourish ourselves to carry out a certain diet.

On many occasions, we realize that something is wrong with our diet. Often because we have a health problem and the doctor has made us aware of it.

Why have a nutritional discipline?

Anything we want to achieve requires effort. Discipline **helps us to act in an orderly manner**, to acquire a habit that is part of our life and with which we can persevere in our purpose.

We usually relate discipline as something imposed, serious, rigorous and boring, even annoying. However, it doesn't have to be that way.

When we find **sufficient motivation** to carry out a plan that helps us achieve our goals, **discipline** becomes a **joyous game that we like to repeat constantly**.

The same thing happens in nutrition. **We need a strategy that motivates and guides us** so that we can achieve our goals.

The advice of a nutritionist establishes the appropriate menus for our physical characteristics and specific circumstances.

But if we lack:

Motivation or willpower, believe that we do not have time to cook or do the shopping, stress overtakes us at that time.

Maybe we need **extra help** to be able to carry out a **balanced diet** successfully. Changing habits is not easy because we cling to the ones we already have without realizing it.

The **nutritional discipline** will provide us with **psychological and dietary tools** to change our eating habits.

To change habits, we need to know which ones are harmful and which ones are healthy. Besides, we also have to **explore ourselves** to discover our mechanical habits since habits are carried out without us being aware of them.

For example, if we are eating meals with bread, we automatically go to the bakery to buy it. We will have to make an effort if, for some reason, we are not going to do it.

It takes **patience, perseverance, and perseverance** to make a change. There are no magic wands or instant formulas. At least not for health. The body and mind have the required time to acquire the eating habits that we have.

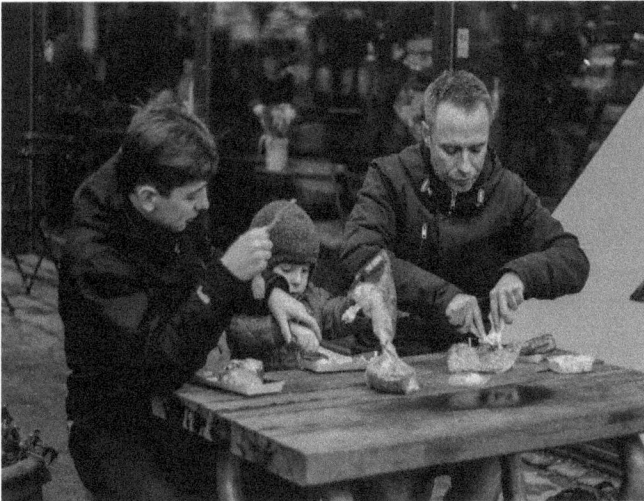

In the same way, it also **takes time** to change them when they harm us. In addition, the social and cultural environment in which we live will greatly influence our possibilities. That is, if your environment is not in tune with your desires for change, you will need much more willpower and motivation to achieve the goal you have set for yourself.

Human beings are social beings. We need to communicate, express ourselves, and share with others what matters to us. We share the good times and those experiences that are more difficult to digest and have left a wound.

All of our relationships influence our character and way of thinking, either positively or negatively. Whether we are or feel alone, we are never completely isolated. And it would not be convenient either, since very few people can endure a state of isolation without getting sick.

When we share our experiences with others, we **transmit information** and, at the same time, **we receive the return** of that information. That is, what others can contribute to us.

The result is that **we feel supported** by the goals we seek and the strategies we propose. Sharing can also serve to modify these strategies, as we can consider the experiences of others.

It **is** always **good to see things from different perspectives**, which can complement ours.

The consequence of **supporting each other is a boost** to that motivation, a boost to our will, and different and complementary strategies with ours.

Practical tips to grasp:

What do you want to achieve with your diet? Some people want to lose weight, but others want to get more energy or improve their health.

Do you compare yourself with someone specific to follow a type of diet? You must be aware of the influence that other people can have on you. Whether they are celebrities that we see on television, advertising, family, or friends. Regardless of your purpose, accept yourself as you are. You will be happier in all aspects.

Get to know yourself thoroughly, your body complexion, health status, and energy needs. You will not require the same energy at 15 as at 40 or 60. Furthermore, each person is different, and if you have any health problems, you have to adapt your diet.

Also, know your character and temperament, attitude, and way of facing different life situations. To achieve success in any goal you set, this aspect is essential. Precisely, you may or may not base on what you think, feel, and believe.

What limits you from getting what you want? What blocks you emotionally and mentally? They are all the "I can't" that you have engraved inside you. As you recognize them, you can gradually transform them into "yes I can" or "yes I could."

Make the changes little by little. Your body has to get used to the new diet. Sudden and rapid changes produce a rebound effect that is demotivating and is often difficult to recover.

Focus on changing only one thing. You don't want to make many changes at once, maybe the goal is too big, and it overwhelms you. It is better to go little by little.

If you have a food addiction that harms you, replace that food with another similar but healthier. Example: industrial pastries for dried fruits, soft drinks for juices.

That your food is varied, full of different colors and flavors.

Eat slowly and enjoy slowly. This way, you counteract stress, and you will be satisfied sooner. So you will need less amount of food.

Share your experiences with others. They may find it helpful, just as the experiences of others can help you.

What you eat affects you mentally

Emotions affect our diet

There is a complex link between food and emotions, so much so that our intestines are often referred to as our second brain since everything we eat can be caused by emotions, and in the same way, our diet can condition our state: psychic and emotional.

Many times we have said that we eat for pleasure. Food has a nutritional function, but eating is pleasant, de-stressing, and therefore, when we feel tired, we can search for food. Little sleep is related to obesity since lack of sleep generates stress, and hormones that increase the desire to eat food are increased in the body.

Similarly, when we are anxious or with emotional problems, we can search for food to feel better. In reality, some foods help calm anxiety because, in their composition, they include tryptophan. This amino acid stimulates the release of serotonin, and it relaxes us at the same time that it makes us happier. These foods are, for example, chocolate, banana, nuts, or yogurt.

Of course, it is normal that we relax and enjoy a pleasant moment, such as eating a chocolate cake from time to time. Still, emotional eating must be controlled because we cannot always eat when we are tired, angry, sad, or happy. Or otherwise, we would end up with excess food. Not everything is solved by eating.

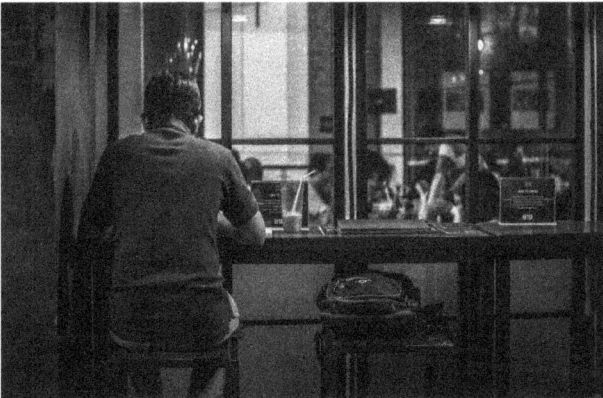

It is also proven that when we eat to calm our emotions, we choose more fatty foods, which can trigger excess fat in the diet, unbalancing it and causing diseases. This is so because our ancestors spent a lot of time without eating and being active, which is stressful. Their body was genetically adapted so that when they had food, they strategically chose the most energy-focused nutrients such as fats. So, fats are associated with a decrease in stress in our brain. Therefore, when we are very tired, a cake with cream may reduce stress more than an apple.

Another proof that emotions affect our diet is that when we are sad, we do not have enough food, or when we eat nervously, we do not like the food. And in extreme cases, emotions can negatively affect digestion, causing irritable bowel syndrome that subsequently conditions the diet's quality.

On the positive side of this link is our emotional history. We often base our preferences or food choices on our emotions in the past. For example, in my case, I love pasta because I associate it with my grandfather and the emotional bond that existed between us. Likewise, a person may prefer a certain food because it reminds them of pleasant emotional moments or rejects a preparation because it is mentally associated with an ugly memory.

Diet affects our emotions

Food and emotions are closely linked, and that is demonstrated by the fact that eating a sweet, we usually feel more relaxed and better. We have also said that there are foods that stimulate serotonin release that helps us better feel.

On the other hand, a healthy diet helps us feel good because many nerve terminals send information to the brain in the intestine. Therefore, preventing intestinal disorders and eating a good quality diet helps us keep under control the emotions. Eating a sufficient diet in micronutrients, with a good amount of soluble fiber, probiotics, and water, is pampering to our digestive system and the organism's second brain.

In the opposite of this complex relationship, we can say that a poor diet can cause depression, so much so that it is known that a diet low in antioxidants, rich in trans fats, and low in micronutrients can give rise to an altered emotional state.

A diet rich in fat throws our biological clock out of control, preventing adequate sleep, which is known to cause stress and emotional distress. As we can see, there is a closed circle that links food with emotions.

It is a dynamic relationship since both foods affect our emotions and vice versa. For our health to be the one that obtains the greatest benefit from this relationship, clearly neither should predominate over the other, but there must be a balance.

So that food is not purely emotional, that is so that the cause of our intake is not always found in emotions but rather that our food consumption is more adjusted to real hunger, we must understand that food provides pleasure and is a de-stressor, but it does not solve our problems and only temporarily calms anxiety.

Suppose we are distressed and look for food. In that case, we think it will not be the solution to this emotion, but that we can resort to other pleasant activities that do not involve food consumption such as reading, listening to music, walking, talking with a friend, among others.

If we let our body enter food before each emotion, we will have an excess of calories that can trigger obesity in the long term.

But if, on the other hand, we repress our desire to eat something sweet from time to time, we will also be altering the balance between emotions and food because when we finally allow ourselves to eat a cake, we will not enjoy it. After eating it, we will feel guilt for having done it, when it is normal to feel pleasure from a little sweet.

So, to establish a balance that does not harm our health, we must control eating our emotions. At the same time, we must allow ourselves from time to time to eat for pleasure, enjoying a tasty and emotional preparation, but if we make this act habitual that links emotions and food, we can fall into a cycle harmful to the body.

Now It Continues

If you are reading this, you reached the end of this book. And I applaud you for making the effort, choice, and finding the will to #MakeTheShift.

I want to thank all my peers, the most prominent researchers I consulted and talked during the past year to get the most classified information on plant-based diet, microbiota, gut health, and optimum nutrition.

I leave you with a gift, the gift of nutrition and the realization that we must act now and make real efforts in progress. We must aspire for a sustainable world, starting ourselves, starting with what we put in our system.

It doesn't stop here and we have a long fight ahead, before we can lay our arms. So, trust your gut, while taking care of your gut and choose plant-based. Always.

Finally, if you enjoyed this book, please let me know your thoughts with a short review on Amazon. All that you need to do is to click the blue link next to the yellow stars that says "customer reviews." You'll then see a gray button that says "Write a customer review"—click that and you're good to go. It means a lot, thank you!

Edyth

www.ingramcontent.com/pod-product-compliance
Lightning Source LLC
Chambersburg PA
CBHW042248040426
42336CB00043B/3361